A PICTURE OF HEALTH

strategies for health education

key stage 3

Gay Gray and Heather Hyde

Illustrated by Pat Murray

Judy Whitmarsh.

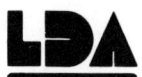

A Picture of Health
LD 664
ISBN 1 85503 146 9
© Gay Gray, Heather Hyde
© illustration Pat Murray
All rights reserved
First published 1992

LDA, Duke Street, Wisbech, Cambs, PE13 2AE

Contents

Acknowledgements — iv

Introduction — 1

ACTIVITY SECTIONS

1. Psychological aspects of health — 17
2. Environmental aspects of health — 41
3. Sex education — 69
4. Family life education — 97
5. Safety — 115
6. Substance use and misuse — 145
7. Food and nutrition — 163
8. Health-related exercise — 191
9. Personal hygiene — 215

Resources — 228

Acknowledgements

To paraphrase the words of Reginald Perrin's boss, 'We wouldn't have got where we are today . . .' without the contact which we have had with teachers and health educators over the years. Our thanks to the many people with whom we have worked, and also to friends in the teaching profession who have suggested creative ways of engaging students in health education.

Particular thanks to Sheila Walden, for keeping us up to date with the effects of current developments in her school.

We are grateful for Elizabeth Longland's secretarial support and care.

Finally, a special thank you to our families. They offered us encouragement and practical support throughout. We would have been struggling without Peter's computer skills and Phil's medical expertise. In the weeks before handing over the manuscript, they put up with our total absorption with the task to the exclusion of all else!

Introduction

Background

> In these closing years of the twentieth century, the path to good health for the people of the world is as bright with promise as it is stormy with challenges. In the face of those challenges, few things we can do today and in the future to promote and protect health have more to offer than health education: this holds true in every part of the world.
>
> (A position paper on health education, by the Director, Division of World Health Organization, and the President, International Union for Health Education, 1991)

One of the major concerns of any society is the health of individuals within it. In 1991, the government published a consultative document on a national strategy for England. Called 'The Health of the Nation', it aims to improve the span of healthy life for the population. Many of the priority areas for development identified are consistent with those set out in the strategic plans of the Health Education Authority, the national organisation which has responsibility for health education in England. All are agreed that education has a vital role to play.

But what responsibility should schools carry, when there are already pressures on the curriculum from many sources?

The Education Reform Act 1988 requires:

> A broadly based curriculum which:
> a) promotes the spiritual, moral, cultural, mental and physical development of pupils at the school and
> b) prepares pupils for the opportunities, responsibilities and experiences of adult life.

The National Curriculum Council (NCC) identified health education as one of the cross-curricular themes which promote the aims in Section 1 of the Act and are an essential part of the curriculum. Health education cannot be left to chance.

Guidelines on health education are given in the publication *Curriculum Guidance 5: Health Education* (NCC, 1990), which identifies nine major components of a health education curriculum for schools. These are:

- Substance use and misuse
- Sex education
- Family life education

Introduction

- Safety
- Health-related exercise
- Food, nutrition
- Personal hygiene
- Environmental aspects of health
- Psychological aspects of health.

The guidelines also lay down appropriate areas of study in each of the components, outlining the knowledge, skills and attitudes to be acquired by students for each key stage.

Health education is expected to contribute to the National Curriculum subject areas – that is English, mathematics, science and technology – through the programmes of study. There are also overlaps with the other cross-curricular themes named by the NCC: economic and industrial understanding, careers education, education for citizenship and environmental education.

This provides schools with starting points for their work in health education, but the problem of how to do it in the classroom still remains.

Purpose of the book

In writing this book we have taken a holistic view of health, understanding it to encompass mental, social, emotional and spiritual health as well as physical health. Our aim is to help students develop their self-esteem, knowledge and skills in order to make positive health choices, and to enable them to act individually and collectively to improve health.

This book offers practical suggestions for health education activities. These are appropriate for Key Stage 3, covering the suggested areas of study for all nine components of the health education curriculum for schools as suggested in *Curriculum Guidance 5*. It has been written to help teachers:

1. to identify the health issues of importance to young people aged 12–14
2. to have access to a range of activities which help young people to identify and develop the skills and knowledge they need, related to these health issues
3. to provide experiences which involve students in their own learning
4. to clarify the health education component of personal and social education (PSE), its cross-curricular nature and its relationship to other subject areas in the National Curriculum.

Before you start

There is often confusion over the meaning of 'health' and the aims of health education. Those involved in health education in schools need to have clarified what they are trying to achieve and to be clear about their motives for involvement, as this will affect what they do and how they work with young people.

What are the things to consider?

INTRODUCTION

School policy

As a teacher starting this work, are you aware of the school's policy towards health education and in particular sex education?

School health education policy begins with the head teacher and the governing body. It should be developed as a result of staff working together and consulting with parents, the local education authority (LEA) and the wider community. Governors and health professionals in the community can be useful sources of advice. It can also be helpful to refer to existing LEA policies such as those on sex education or drug education.

It should be noted that at LEA level, schools are strongly advised to draw up a policy on drug and alcohol education. Moreover, the National Curriculum Science Order requires governing bodies to be responsible for determining schools' policies on the organisation and content of sex education. It is their duty (under Section 18(2) of the Education (No 2) Act 1986):

> – (a) to consider separately (while having regard to the local education authority's statement under section 17 of this Act on their policy in relation to the secular curriculum in maintained schools) the question whether sex education should form part of the secular curriculum for the school; and

> – (b) to make and keep up to date a separate written statement of their policy with regard to the content and organisation of the relevant part of the curriculum; or where they conclude that sex education should not form part of the secular curriculum, of that conclusion.

Section 46 of the Act requires that:

> The local education authority by whom any county, voluntary or special school is maintained, and the governing body and the head teacher of the school, shall take such steps as are reasonably practicable to secure that where sex education is given to any pupils at the school it is given in such a manner as to encourage those pupils to have due regard to moral considerations and the value of family life.

A school policy should be consistent with national and local guidelines. It needs to be approached at two levels: a commitment to promoting the health of all staff and students who work in the school and a specific commitment to teach health issues in a planned way. It should make clear where health education is located in the whole curriculum, how it is taught and the ways in which healthy behaviour is being promoted. Working documents, which accept the need for review and change in policy, will encourage staff support and debate.

Co-ordination of health education is best undertaken by a key member of staff with sufficient status and appropriate skills.

How can it be organised?

The majority of secondary schools offer some form of health education to their students. There are several ways in which this can be timetabled and some schools may choose to use different combinations at different key stages. The models set out below will be familiar to many schools and are taken from *Curriculum Guidance 5*.

PERMEATING THE WHOLE CURRICULUM
Positive:

- Secures a place for health within the statutory curriculum
- Ensures all teachers take some responsibility for aspects of their work

Negative:

- May be difficult to incorporate appropriate teaching and learning methods
- May be seen as a peripheral element within the subject
- May be difficult to deal adequately with sensitive issues
- May be difficult to co-ordinate a theme that lacks sharp definition

AS A SEPARATELY TIMETABLED SUBJECT
Positive:

- Secures a place in the curriculum for health education
- Likely to be taught by specialists
- Facilitates progression and continuity

Negative:

- May focus on cognitive aspects, ignoring work relating to attitudes and behaviour
- Difficult to find space in the crowded curriculum
- Isolates health education from other elements of the curriculum

AS PART OF A PSE COURSE
Positive:

- Has the potential to be taught by a special team
- Allows links to be established between health education and the other cross-curricular themes
- Facilitates progression and continuity

Negative:

- Competition between cross-curricular themes may be restricting
- May become isolated from other elements of the whole curriculum

AS PART OF A PASTORAL/TUTORIAL PROGRAMME
Positive:

- Most teachers will have some responsibility for health education
- Teachers are in touch with the needs and emotional development of students within their care

Introduction

Negative:
- Routine tasks may leave little time for health education
- Teachers may be reluctant to teach about health matters, particularly the sensitive issues

In Key Stage 3 many schools teach health education through subjects such as science. However, it is important that the physical, mental, emotional and social aspects of any health topic are included. For example, in learning about the reproductive system, the wider aspects of sexuality and personal relationships should be covered. This may be difficult to include in the science curriculum, especially with the added pressure of meeting the requirements of the National Curriculum.

Many schools overcome the problem of breadth by providing a timetabled PSE course which builds on the learning acquired elsewhere. This gives students an opportunity to practise skills and clarify attitudes, values and beliefs.

How does this book support the National Curriculum?

The NCC identified nine major components of the cross-curricular theme of health education. These form the framework of this book.

It is important to consider how these nine components could contribute to the whole curriculum. Many of the activities in the book could contribute to programmes of study leading to levels of attainment for Key Stage 3 in the foundation subjects. Where these are available, we have referenced them in the summary chart at the end of this section. At the time of writing, Statutory Orders have been published for mathematics, English, science and technology, although these are still under review.

The attainment targets identified in the summary chart are:

Science
Attainment Target (1991) 1   Scientific investigation
Attainment Target (1991) 2   Life and living processes

English
Attainment Target 1   Speaking and listening
Attainment Target 2   Reading
Attainment Target 3   Writing
Attainment Target 4/5   Presentation

Mathematics
Attainment Target 1   Using and applying mathematics
Attainment Target 5   Handling data

Technology
Attainment Target 1   Identifying needs and opportunities
Attainment Target 4   Evaluating

The summary also shows the links between the activities and the other cross-curricular themes of PSE, namely: economic and industrial understanding, career education and guidance, education for citizenship and environmental education.

INTRODUCTION

Where should I start?

One criticism which young people often have of health education is that they feel they are being preached at, that it's about what not to do! To be effective it must be interactive, with students being active participants rather than passive recipients. This means involving them from the start, finding out what they are bringing in terms of experience and knowledge, so that together you can identify future needs.

Each young person in their early teens will bring the sum of their life experiences to that point. They will have been influenced by the culture in which they have been brought up. Some will have learnt the skills of adapting to two different cultures, one at home with their family and one at school and in the wider community. They will be at varying stages of development, with some not yet starting puberty and others perhaps being sexually active. If you make assumptions about their needs, you could be completely off the mark.

They will have picked up information over the years from a range of sources, including parents, the media, friends and previous schooling. Some of that information may be incorrect. There may be gaps in their knowledge. They may be more knowledgeable than you over certain issues! Once you have discovered their level of knowledge and perceptions of health, it becomes easier to select appropriate activities.

Similarly, it is important to communicate in words that all parties understand. To give an example, an AIDS worker was asked to a youth club one evening to run a session for the club members. She gave a rather formal input about the way in which HIV was transmitted, talking about it being spread through semen. The youth worker noticed one boy getting very agitated and asked him later what the matter was. The reply? 'These seamen make me sick. I've a good mind to go down to the docks and bash a few.' We need to keep checking that the lines of communication are clear.

Two of the main requirements for anyone teaching health education are a genuine interest in young people and a willingness to listen to what they have to say and to value their experience. One of the easiest ways to identify their needs is to ask them! Sessions which involve asking them to discuss in small groups what they want to get from a health education programme (and what they definitely do not want!), what particularly interests them, what they want to know and what skills they want to develop can be very useful. However, you may find that simply asking them 'cold', with no warm-up discussion, leads to sparse results. You need some form of activity or stimulus material to trigger discussion.

Activities which work well include **brainstorming**, to discover what they already know and words they might use; **photographs**, to discuss perceptions; **quizzes**, to explore existing knowledge and identify what else they would like to know; and **collages and drawings**, to encourage expression. Most of the activities in this book involve encouraging students to work and discuss in small groups, and to listen to one another. The teacher's skill is in drawing out the learning.

For many young people, who tend to perceive health education as 'finger wagging' and 'victim blaming', an approach which begins by considering wider social issues may be appropriate. Rather than focusing on the individual (eg why people should not smoke), look at the context within which that individual operates (eg the ways in which tobacco companies market their products).

Encourage them to carry out surveys into the facilities available in the community and to suggest ways forward to meet the needs of people in their community.

Identifying their needs is not something which happens at the beginning and then stops. It is a process which underpins health education. It is a continual questioning and reflecting on what is appropriate, on what they have learnt and what they need to do next.

Planning a programme

If you do all the activities in this book, you will have covered the appropriate areas of study described in *Curriculum Guidance 5*.

However, if you are working in a person-centred way, your sense of direction and organisation of a programme must reflect the needs of the people you are working with. Therein lies the dilemma! Will you be bound by a syllabus, or open to responding to the needs of the group? In reality, there will probably be a combination of the two, taking in certain ground which you think it important to cover, but staying as flexible as possible in order to meet students' needs.

If you are to work in an experiential way, encouraging students to take responsibility for their own learning, you will need to engage in a cycle of learning. The experiential learning model developed by David Kolb is illustrated below.

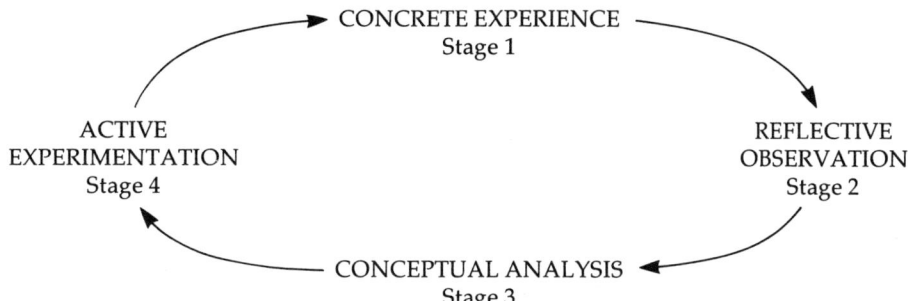

Stage 1 involves the students having a concrete experience or activity. This might be a quiz, a game, a role play, an outing, a survey. The list is endless! Using the example of a role play on resisting pressure, Stage 1 could involve students working in pairs, to practise saying 'No'.

The next stage (Stage 2, reflective observation) allows them time to reflect on that experience. Where the role play is concerned, students would discuss in their pairs how they felt during the role play: what worked, what didn't work, what behaviour helped or hindered. This reflection could then be shared in the whole group.

Stage 3, conceptual analysis, involves drawing out the general learning from the activity. To go back to our example, you would encourage them to see what general concepts they can draw from their experience in the role play. Typical questions would be: If they did 'A' in real life, would

Introduction

'B' tend to happen? Do girls/boys generally behave like that? How would other people react? What would make it easy or difficult to resist pressure?

To highlight the importance which we attach to this stage, we have included a *processing questions* section in each activity to help teachers to draw out the learning. These questions are crucial. Without them, students could be left thinking, 'OK. That was interesting ... but so what?'

Stage 4, active experimentation, involves forward planning, deciding on how they are going to use what they have learnt, what they are going to try out in life. It may involve practising the skill of saying 'No' at home, or at the youth club. As a result of that experience, together you will be able to identify future learning needs ... which takes you back to Stage 1.

The main focus of working in this way is the person and her/his experience.

Group work

If students are to be encouraged to discuss their own feelings and share their views on a wide range of issues including relationships, teachers need to encourage the development of a safe, supportive environment in the classroom. This means creating a climate where people value one another's contributions, listen to one another and are sensitive to the feelings of others. As the group evolves, you may find this could be helped by encouraging students to put down in writing ground rules for the group. It is important then to monitor their effectiveness, and to apply them.

An essential element of health education is helping students to develop relationship skills, and to learn how to be effective members of a group. The skills required of a teacher are those of working with groups and facilitating their development. They need not be the fount of all wisdom. If students want up-to-date information, a teacher needs to know how to help them access it, via written materials and agencies in the community, for example.

Besides a willingness to listen, teachers will need to have at their fingertips a wide range of approaches to encourage involvement in the group. It was with this in mind that we wrote the book, intending that teachers should select activities to suit their groups, in their various stages of development, rather than following through the book from the start to the finish.

At the end of each activity we indicate posible follow-up work, showing links with other activities in the book and with other subject areas.

Evaluation

Evaluation is a way to monitor your progress – have you achieved what you set out to do? It involves being clear about why you are evaluating something and what it is you want to know. Evaluation is not the same as assessment. Many activities in the book are quizzes and question-

Introduction

naires and these can help you to assess the level of students' knowledge. Assessment is only part of evaluation.

Evaluation can be a means of understanding the needs of your students; an example is asking them to identify what they would like to learn or know more about, and what skills they would like to develop further. It can be a way of gaining students' reactions to a lesson, for example by using a simple review sheet.

Students can be encouraged to evaluate their own performance, for example how well they participated in a group, or what support they gave each other. Teachers will draw up their own questions appropriate to the group and the lessons being evaluated.

Evaluation is a way of reflecting on how effective you are as a teacher and of deciding how to improve a learning situation. Questions you might ask yourself are:

- Did you make the purpose of the lesson clear to students?
- Were your instructions clear?
- Did you draw upon students' experiences?
- How did the lesson relate to what had gone before?

Evaluation is a continuous process which helps you to adjust your planning to meet the needs of your group.

Timing

For each activity in the book, we have given an indication of the amount of time an activity should take. However, this can only be an approximation as it will vary depending on the group.

Summary of activities

The following chart shows you at a glance the content and aims of all the activities and how they can contribute to learning in other areas of the National Curriculum.

Activity	Purpose	National Curriculum links
SECTION 1: PSYCHOLOGICAL ASPECTS OF HEALTH		
1 **Who am I?** Collage/drawing	Getting to know one another	English AT1 Careers
2 **Identifying personal qualities and strengths** 'Things that describe me'	Clarifying self-image and building self-confidence	English AT1 Careers
3 **Warm or cold?** Interview, montage	Exploring put-downs and positive comments	English AT1

INTRODUCTION

	Activity	Purpose	National Curriculum links
4	**The picture of youth in the media** Collage	Demonstrating ways in which media portray young people	English AT2 Citizenship
5	**A story** Story, exercise	Challenging stereotypes	English AT2 Citizenship
6	**Everyone is unique** Photographs	Encouraging positive attitude towards move to adulthood	English AT1 Science AT2 Careers
7	**Body image** Advertisements	Understanding wide range of normality in body shape	English AT2 Science AT2
8	**Recognising emotions in yourself and others** Situations, vocabulary, mime	Recognising and expressing feelings	English AT1 Careers
9	**The meaning of assertiveness** Situations	Exploring assertive, aggressive and passive behaviours	English AT1 Careers
10	**Being assertive** Role play	Practising being assertive	English AT1 Careers
11	**Positive strokes** Writing on cards	Practising giving and receiving praise	English AT1 Careers
SECTION 2: ENVIRONMENTAL ASPECTS OF HEALTH			
12	**What is a healthy person?** Statements	Exploring what is meant by health	English AT1 Science AT2 Environment
13	**Influences on health** Scenarios	Identifying positive and negative influences	English AT1, 2 & 3 Science AT2 Technology AT1 Careers Economic and industrial understanding Environment
14	**Infectious/non-infectious diseases** Spot the difference exercise	Distinguishing between infectious/non-infectious diseases	Science AT2 Environment
15	**Card sort** Card game	Understanding causes, spread and prevention of infectious diseases	Science AT2 Environment

Introduction

Activity	Purpose	National Curriculum links
16 **Where to go for help** Problem and solution cards	Informing about range of services and help available	English AT1 & 3 Careers Citizenship Environment
17 **A visit to the doctor** Reflection on personal experience	Identifying and practising skills needed to visit doctor	English AT1 Careers Environment
18 **The influence of the media and advertising** Analysis and decoding sheet	Understanding techniques used to promote products	English AT2 Economic and industrial understanding Environment
19 **Attitudes to the environment** Questionnaire	Exploring attitudes to the environment	English AT1 Technology AT1 Citizenship Environment
20 **A healthy community** Checklist, mapping exercise	Learning what makes a healthy community	English AT4 & 5 Technology AT1 Citizenship Environment

SECTION 3: SEX EDUCATION

21 **Me as a member of a group** Brainstorm	Exploring benefits and disadvantages of group membership	English AT1 Careers Citizenship
22 **Friends** Diamond nine exercise	Identifying qualities looked for in a friend	English AT1
23 **Listening skills** Listening in pairs	Understanding and practising listening	English AT1 Careers
24 **Where do I stand?** Continuum	Exploring attitudes on relationships and sexuality	English AT1 Careers Citizenship
25 **Different values** Stories	Discussing and exploring moral values	English AT1 & 2 Careers Citizenship
26 **Assumptions** Drawing of man and woman	Exploring stereotypes of men and women	English AT1 Careers Citizenship
27 **Love songs** Tape	Exploring views on love and sex	English AT1
28 **Problem pages** Letters from magazines/comics	Discussing relationship problems	English AT1

Introduction

Activity	Purpose	National Curriculum links
29 **Who'd fall for that line?** Common 'lines' exercise	Resisting pressure into sexual activity	English AT1 Citizenship
30 **What's in a word?** Brainstorm	Exploring words used in talking about sex	English AT1
31 **Is it true?** Quiz	Providing accurate information about sexual issues	Science AT2
32 **Contraception** Leaflets, articles	Identifying ways of finding information about contraception	Science AT2
33 **Using a condom** Card sort	Increasing awareness about correct use of condoms	

SECTION 4: FAMILY LIFE EDUCATION

Activity	Purpose	National Curriculum links
34 **Family roles** Brainstorm, cartoons,	Examining different roles and behaviour patterns in family	English AT1 Citizenship
35 **The trouble with grown-ups** Questionnaire	Identifying ways of solving family conflict	English AT1 Careers Citizenship
36 **Changes** Timeline	Considering what helps or hinders coping with change	English AT1 Careers Citizenship
37 **The needs of children** Pairs, photographs	Developing work on needs of children	English AT1 Science AT2 Citizenship
38 **Coping with loss** Photographs, circle of feelings	Understanding and coping with loss	English AT1 Careers Citizenship
39 **Looking after children** Visitors	Recognising factors involved in planning and having a family	English AT1 Careers Citizenship
40 **Early learning** Age cards	Understanding what is involved in looking after children	English AT1 Science AT2 Technology AT1 Careers Citizenship

SECTION 5: SAFETY

Activity	Purpose	National Curriculum links
41 **Are you a risk-taker?** Questionnaire	Exploring positive and negative aspects of risk-taking	English AT1 Careers

Introduction

Activity	Purpose	National Curriculum links
42 **What are the chances?** Risk factor game	Influence of risk factors on diseases and health	Mathematics AT5 Science AT1
43 **Decisions, decisions** 'How do you decide?'	Promoting and practising decision-making	English AT1 Careers
44 **Who is responsible?** Role play	Considering responsibility for safety in public places	English AT1 & 4/5 Technology AT1 Citizenship Economic and industrial understanding Environment
45 **Keeping safe** Situation cards	Analysing and assessing situations of safety	English AT1 & 4/5 Environment
46 **Accidents do happen** Knowledge quiz	Increasing awareness of causes of accidents and what to do in emergencies	Mathematics AT5 Citizenship Environment
47 **Bullying** Scenarios	Coping with bullying	English AT1 Citizenship
48 **Vandalism** Articles, photographs, drawing, jigsaw	Exploring perceptions of vandalism and what to do about it	English AT1 Technology AT4 Citizenship Environment

SECTION 6: SUBSTANCE USE AND MISUSE

49 **Alphabetical brainstorm** Brainstorm	Exploring knowledge about drugs	English AT1 Citizenship
50 **Types of drugs** Matching exercise	Providing information about different types of drugs	Science AT2
51 **Is it OK?** Continuum	Examining attitudes and social acceptability of drugs	English AT1 Citizenship
52 **Why do people take drugs?** People cards	Exploring why people take drugs	English AT1 Citizenship Environment
53 **The effects of drugs** Quiz	Providing information about the effects of drug-taking	Science AT2 Citizenship
54 **Carousel** Role play	Identifying how to refuse drugs	English AT1

Introduction

Activity	Purpose	National Curriculum links
55 **Do you know what you're taking?** Calculation	Providing information about alcoholic strengths of different drinks	Mathematics AT1
56 **Anti-smoking** Posters	Considering measures to discourage smoking	English AT1 & 2 Citizenship
SECTION 7: FOOD AND NUTRITION		
57 **A healthy appetite** Quiz	Providing a guide to healthy eating	Science AT2
58 **Diet and lifestyles** Card match	Understanding link between diet and lifestyle	Science AT2 Citizenship Economic and industrial understanding Environment
59 **Food handling** Photographs, pictures, checklist	Raising awareness of need for food hygiene	Science AT2 Technology AT1 Environment
60 **Do you know what you're eating?** Food labels/ cardsort	Understanding what is in food	English AT2 Mathematics AT5 Science AT1 Citizenship Economic and industrial understanding Environment
61 **Junk food** Personal eating profiles	Recognising eating patterns and identifying how to change them	English AT1 Technology AT4 Economic and industrial understanding Environment
62 **What's right for me?** Personal plan	Understanding link between food intake and energy output	Science AT2
63 **I can't refuse** Strategies for positive self-talk	Practising positive self-talk	English AT1 Careers
64 **A school survey** Survey, interviews	Enquiring into school meals service	English AT1 & 4/5 Citizenship Environment
SECTION 8: HEALTH-RELATED EXERCISE		
65 **Why exercise?** Quotes from young people	Discussing reasons for exercising	English AT1 Citizenship

Introduction

	Activity	Purpose	National Curriculum links
66	**There's more than one way** Brainstorm, stars	Considering appropriateness of types of exercise/sport for different people	Science AT2 Citizenship Environment
67	**What is there to do?** Research project	Investigating sports facilities in the community	English AT4/5 Mathematics AT5 Technology AT1 Citizenship Environment
68	**Taking your pulse rate** Practical activity	Learning how to monitor pulse rate	Science AT1
69	**How fit are you?** Exercise diary, fitness tests	Increasing awareness of fitness and value of exercise	Mathematics AT1 Science AT1
70	**Choosing what's right for you** Action plan, contracting in pairs	Deciding on action plan	English AT1 Careers
71	**What's stopping you?** Matching exercise, devising case-studies	Identifying strategies for overcoming resistance to exercising	English AT1 Citizenship
72	**A stressful wordsearch** Wordsearch	Discussing ways of preventing stress	English AT4
73	**Learning to relax** Techniques	Demonstrating simple relaxation techniques	

SECTION 9: PERSONAL HYGIENE

	Activity	Purpose	National Curriculum links
74	**The hygiene game** Creating game	Considering personal hygiene issues for different age groups	English AT4/5 Science AT2 Technology AT1 & 2
75	**Problems** Problem pages	Finding answers to hygiene problems	English AT3
76	**What do I really need?** Collage	Discussion of hygiene products	
77	**Keeping clean** Pictures/ photographs	Exploring constraints on keeping clean	English AT1 Citizenship Environment
78	**Counting the cost** Research project	Considering the cost of keeping clean	Mathematics AT5 Science AT1 Economics

SECTION 1

Psychological aspects of health

SECTION 1: PSYCHOLOGICAL ASPECTS OF HEALTH

ACTIVITY 1: *Who am I?*

Purpose
- To help students to share something about themselves
- To help them to know each other
- To encourage creative expression
- To encourage group-building

Time needed 30 minutes

What you need Large sheets of paper/card. Glue. Scissors. Coloured felt-tip pens. Selection of magazines.

How you do it

1. Explain that they are to make a collage or drawing that will give other people some idea of who they are. They may want to show their interests, or what is important to them, or things they like or dislike – the choice is theirs. Similarly, how they do it is up to them. Explain that there is a range of materials to help with this. They can cut pictures from magazines or draw. They may want to use symbols or words. Give each person a large sheet of paper. Allow 10 minutes.
2. Ask them to join with three others. Each person in turn shares what they have done.
3. As a group they are to try to find something that they all have in common.
4. Bring the group together and encourage discussion.

Variation

Before the lesson, prepare the sheets of paper/card so that they will eventually fit together in some way. This might be as sections of a jigsaw, petals of a flower or sections of a wheel. Code the sheets by marking the back with a coloured dot or a certain word. Once they have completed their collage, they should find the people with a similar code to themselves, form a small group and share.

Processing questions
- Did they find it easy or difficult to identify something in common?
- If they managed to do that, what was it?
- Was it easy to create a collage?
- Did it help in getting to know people?

SECTION 1: PSYCHOLOGICAL ASPECTS OF HEALTH

ACTIVITY 2
Identifying personal qualities and strengths

Purpose
- To help students to clarify their self-image and build their self-confidence
- To encourage listening skills and support for each other

Time needed 30 minutes

What you need A copy of Activity Sheet 2 for each student. Pens.

How you do it
1. Give each student a copy of Activity Sheet 2. Ask them to close their eyes and think about words or phrases that describe things that they like about themselves, qualities they have or things they can do.
2. Ask each student to write at least six words or phrases on the sheet in the space provided. There are some words and phrases already on the sheet to act as prompts.
3. Ask each student to choose a partner to work with. They should take it in turns to describe themselves to each other, sharing the things that they like most about themselves. The partner should try to show that s/he is listening carefully without interrupting.
4. After each partner has shared her/his list, ask each pair to discuss if there are things that they would like to change about themselves. How might they go about this?

Processing questions
- Was it easy to identify qualities and skills in yourself?
- How comfortable do we feel when talking about things we are good at?
- How easy was it to listen without interrupting?
- How did it feel to be listened to?

Suggestions for follow-up work Activities 9 and 10 on assertiveness, Activity 23 on listening skills and Activity 11 on giving and receiving praise.

SECTION 1: PSYCHOLOGICAL ASPECTS OF HEALTH

ACTIVITY SHEET 2 — 'Things that describe me'

Prompt words | **My list**

I AM   fun   ....

a good listener   ....

relaxed   ....

confident   ....

kind   ....

healthy   ....

good-looking   ....

generous   ....

a good swimmer   ....

sympathetic   ....

THINGS I LIKE BEST ABOUT MYSELF   ....

SKILLS I WOULD LIKE TO DEVELOP   ....

HOW I MIGHT GO ABOUT IT   ....

This sheet is only for your own use. You choose what you wish to share with your partner.

SECTION 1: PSYCHOLOGICAL ASPECTS OF HEALTH

ACTIVITY 3

Warm or cold?

Purpose	• To explore how students' self-esteem is affected by other people's words and actions
	• To begin to identify ways of coping with this
Time needed	40 minutes
What you need	Eight pieces of card for each group of four: four in the shape of grey clouds, and four in the shape of yellow suns (with an optional smiling face!). Blutack. Felt-tip pens.
How you do it	1 Point out to students that how we feel about ourselves is often affected by how people treat us. Each time we hear something good about ourselves or someone shows us they care, we tend to feel better. You could say that a particular person has given us a warm, sunny feeling. Each time we are put down, ridiculed, rejected or criticised, we tend to feel worse, to feel 'put down'. Give students some examples of 'put-downs', such as 'You're stupid' or 'Don't you even know that?' Ask them for other examples.
	2 Ask them, in pairs, to interview one another for 5 minutes each about a recent time when they felt put down and then a time when someone helped them to feel warm and good about themselves . . . it may have been with a hug, or a friendly smile, or by something they said.
	3 Invite each pair to join with another. Give each foursome four cloud cards and four sun cards. They should write, in large letters, on each of the cloud cards one way in which people can put them down and make them feel small, and on each sun card a way in which people can help them to feel better about themselves.
	4 Make a cloudy sky on one wall. Ask each group to put up their clouds, reading them out as they do so, and grouping them so that similar ones are together. Encourage them to listen to one another's contributions and to check what was meant by the words on each cloud.
	5 Repeat the process with the suns, either building a separate sunny sky or covering the clouds.
Processing questions	• Which cards were the easiest/most difficult to write?
	• Why do people put others down?
	• Are there any ways in which we put ourselves down (eg taking more notice of criticism than compliments)?
	• How can we make sure in this group that we help people to feel good about themselves?

Suggestions for follow-up work

- Ask them to do some detective work. For one day they should record any put-downs that they hear at school and at home. How did people tend to react? Suggest a reason why each put-down was made in the first place. Get them to report their findings at a later session.
- Contract with the group to try to avoid putting one another down for a day/week and build in a review session of how successful they were.
- This could lead into a session where the group establishes ground rules for working together in future.

SECTION 1: PSYCHOLOGICAL ASPECTS OF HEALTH

ACTIVITY 4: The picture of youth in the media

Purpose To demonstate the way that the media portray young people

Time needed 30 minutes

What you need Newspapers. Magazines. Journals. Scissors. Glue. Flipchart paper. Coloured felt-tip pens.

How you do it
1. Divide the group into small groups of three to five.
2. Provide each group with newspapers, magazines and journals. Ask each group to mark, or cut out, any articles or stories about young people. They could make a collage of the examples they found.
3. Encourage them to examine the collages and to look at the use of language in reporting events (eg how the word 'youth' is used). Get them to consider whether this leads to a stereotyped view of teenage behaviour.

Processing questions
- How many reports refer to the aggressive habits of young people, and how many stories show young people in a positive light?
- Can they find examples of the same story reported in different ways? If so, why do they think this is?
- How realistic is the view of young people shown in the media and press?
- Are there examples of sensational headlines, for example:
  'GANG IN RAMPAGE IN NEW SHOPPING PRECINCT'
  'YOUTHS TERRIFY BUS PASSENGERS'
  'POLICE HUNT YOUTHS AFTER DISTURBANCE AT DISCO'?

Suggestions for follow-up work
- Ask them to compile a newspaper of their own which reports on the positive achievements of young people and which reflects their interests and concerns.
- Repeat the activity using newspapers, magazines and journals to find out how elderly people are represented. How does this relate to the elderly people they know or meet?

SECTION 1: PSYCHOLOGICAL ASPECTS OF HEALTH

ACTIVITY 5 — *A story*

Purpose
- To identify and clarify some of the everyday assumptions people make
- To look at the reasons why they are made
- To get students to begin to challenge stereotypes

Time needed 30 minutes

What you need A copy of Activity Sheet 5 for each student. Pens.

How you do it
1. Hand out copies of Activity Sheet 5. Ask them not to discuss it. Read the story out loud.
2. When the story has been read, ask them to circle their answers to each statement without letting others see their choices.
3. Ask them to compare and tally their responses, working in groups of four.
4. Then read out each statement and ask each group to indicate their scores (the Eurovision Song Contest strikes again!) Ask for volunteers to explain the reason for their choice.
5. Discuss the assumptions that influenced their choices.

Processing questions
- Why do we jump to conclusions?
- Do we tend to read things into different words?
- Is it useful sometimes to make assumptions about people?
- When could it be harmful?

Suggestions for follow-up work
- Ask them to observe and note during the following week common assumptions that they come across. Discuss these at a later session.
- Activity 26, exploring stereotyping by gender, and Activity 52 about drug-taking.

SECTION 1: PSYCHOLOGICAL ASPECTS OF HEALTH

A story

Terry looked forward to Friday and Saturday evenings. Time during the week seemed to go very slowly. Most evenings were spent watching the TV or helping look after the other children in the family, but weekends were different. Terry would meet up with a close friend, Chris, and they would usually go to a local pub or sometimes see a film. Terry's parents were strict, expecting them home early and strongly disapproving of Terry drinking beer. They were not keen on Chris, whom they saw as a bad influence, and likely to get Terry into trouble.

Terry didn't think it was fair. Chris was allowed to stay out late and go to all-night parties. Chris was expected to do well at school, particularly in science, and was being encouraged by one parent to follow the family tradition and become a dentist. The only encouragement that Terry got was 'Doesn't Terry get on well with people? Someone like that will never be lonely.' They didn't seem to worry whether Terry would get a good job or not.

It was difficult to see why Terry and Chris were so fond of one another as they came from such different backgrounds.

Circle your response to each of the following statements

Terry is a girl	True	False	Don't know
Chris is a boy	True	False	Don't know
Terry is over 16	True	False	Don't know
Dentistry is for boys	True	False	Don't know
Terry's parents are poor	True	False	Don't know
Terry and Chris are both girls	True	False	Don't know
Terry and Chris are both boys	True	False	Don't know

SECTION 1: PSYCHOLOGICAL ASPECTS OF HEALTH

ACTIVITY 6
Everyone is unique

Purpose To encourage positive feelings in young people towards the changes they face as they move from childhood to adulthood

Time needed 60 minutes

What you need Photographs of young people at different stages – baby, toddler, primary school age. Copies for each group of Activity Sheet 6, which shows young people of the same age but differing in height, weight and appearance. Flipchart paper, pens.

How you do it
1. Ask students if possible to bring two or three photographs of themselves at different ages. Display these carefully (they may have sentimental value) around the walls. Form the students into pairs and ask them to try to guess who is who in the photographs.
2. Ask groups, working in fours, to brainstorm the changes which children go through either between 0 and 5 years or between 5 and 10 years, using flipchart paper. Encourage them to think about physical changes as well as what children can do.
3. Share the results.
4. Give each group, in the same fours, a copy of Activity Sheet 6. Ask them to answer the questions on the sheet.
5. Get each group to feed back the possible concerns of the young people in the drawing. Ask them to suggest what might help them. Point out that this drawing has frozen a moment in time and that the people in it will continue to change.
6. Get the students to form pairs and take it in turns to interview each other about a change they have been through. (This could be a change of school, a change of friends, moving house.) How did they feel before, during and after the change? What helped them through it?

Suggestions for follow-up work
- They could write a story in which they imagine themselves in ten years' time.
- Ask them to find out how a young person of the same age as themselves would have spent their day fifty years ago and one hundred years ago. Get them to discuss what changes have taken place in the lives of young people.

SECTION 1: PSYCHOLOGICAL ASPECTS OF HEALTH

Everyone is unique

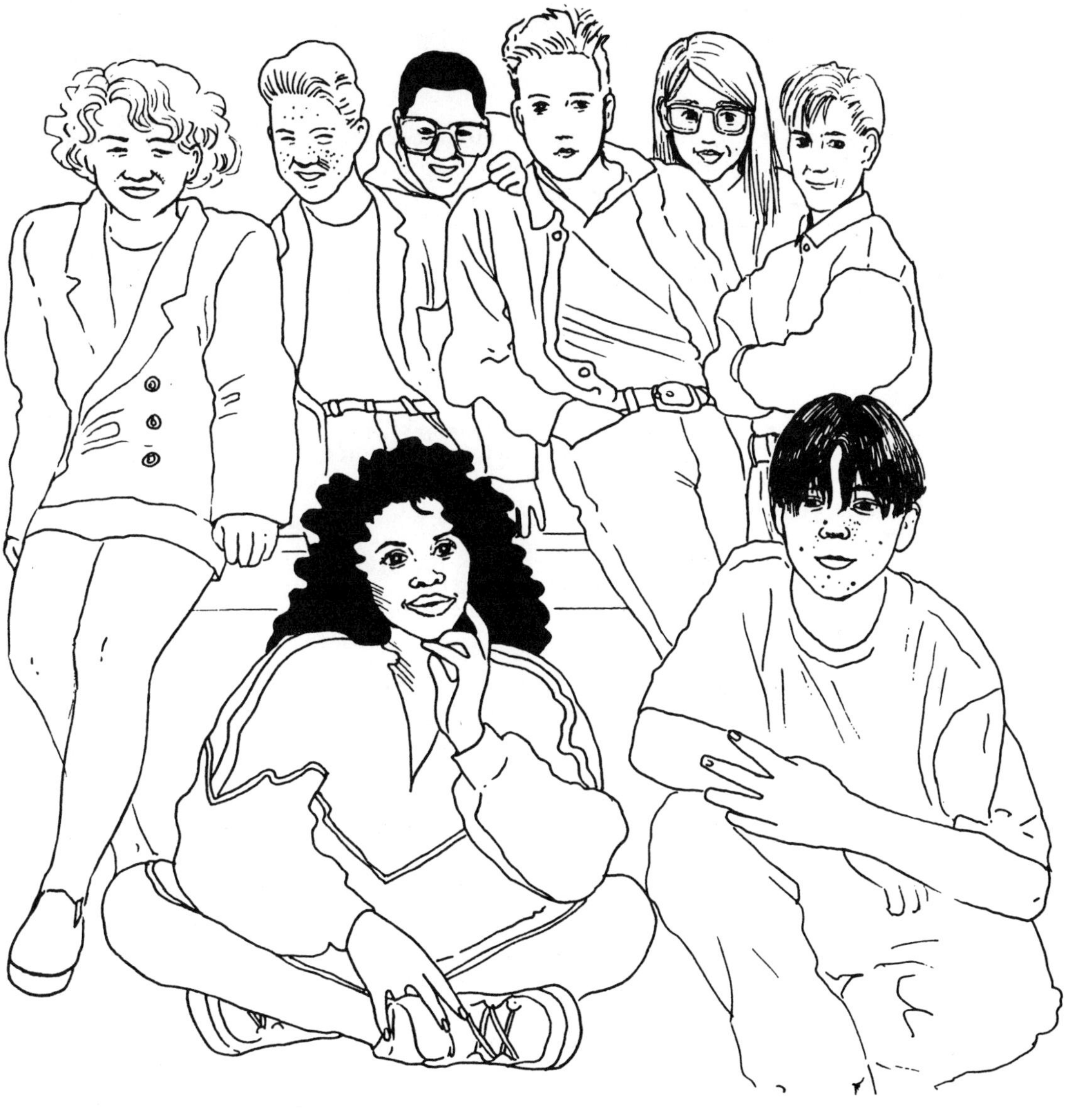

1. Choose one person from the drawing.
2. In pairs, discuss how this person might feel about themself.
3. What concerns might they have about themself?
4. What might help the person to feel good about themself?

Section 1: Psychological Aspects of Health

Activity 7: Body image

Purpose	• To help young people to understand the wide range of normality in adult body shapes of men and women • To counteract stereotyped presentations of masculinity and femininity
Time needed	30 minutes
What you need	A collection of advertisements (with the product name removed) using men's and women's bodies to attract attention. A separate list which gives the names of the products in the advertisements. A collection of pictures of well-known successful men and women who do not conform to media stereotypes. Pictures of people in everyday situations; these could be collected by the students themselves.
How you do it	1. Divide the class into groups of four or five. Give each group a collection of advertisements and ask them to guess the products each is promoting. How do their guesses compare with the list of the products? 2. Encourage the groups to discuss what attracts them to an advertisement. Is it the use of colour? Humour? Famous people such as sports personalities? Is it the use of men's and women's bodies? How real are the images portrayed in the advertisements? Are most women really slim, long limbed and in their early 20s? Are the majority of men tall, broad shouldered and craggy jawed? 3. Ask them what 'hidden messages' advertisements give them about themselves. Do they influence how they see themselves? Can they learn something from the pictures of well-known men and women who do not look like the ideals that appear in the media? 4. Get the students to make a collection of pictures or photographs of people in ordinary situations going about their daily lives. Ask each group to comment on how they compare with the advertisements. 5. Invite each group to make a presentation of what they think makes a person attractive, remembering the qualities they value in a person. Do they put too much emphasis on physical appearance?
Suggestions for follow-up work	• Ask them to find out the 'average' height for men and women in Britain today, and whether this has changed in the last hundred years. • Continue work on the influence of the media, as in Activity 18.

SECTION 1: PSYCHOLOGICAL ASPECTS OF HEALTH

ACTIVITY 8
Recognising emotions in yourself and others

Purpose
- To help students to be aware that we all experience a wide range of feelings
- To help them develop a vocabulary to describe and express feelings
- To explore non-verbal ways of expressing emotions
- To help them to recognise emotions in other people

Time needed 30 minutes

What you need A copy of Activity Sheet 8 for each person. Pens.

How you do it
1. Ask the participants to think about the feelings they would have in the situations printed on Activity Sheet 8.
2. Ask them to list three feelings for each situation. A list of prompt 'feeling words' is given to help.
3. Ask them to share their responses to the situations in groups of three. Were there common feelings? Why do they think it is important to be able to describe their feelings?
4. Choose one of the 'feeling words' from the activity sheet. Each person, in turn, should attempt to mime her/his word to the other two.

Processing questions
- Do people try to hide their feelings?
- How successful were they at guessing the emotions portrayed in the mime?
- What did it feel like if people were unable to guess their mime?
- Is it important to be able to judge how other people are feeling?

Suggestions for follow-up work Get young people to observe the expressions of people in the street. Invite them to make up a story about what they think one of these people might be feeling at the time, and why.

SECTION 1: PSYCHOLOGICAL ASPECTS OF HEALTH

ACTIVITY SHEET 8

'How would I feel if?'

Write down three responses to each situation:

How would I feel if

- My best friend moved to another town?

- I failed a test I worked hard for?

- I had been blamed for something I didn't do?

- I lost my favourite tape?

- My friend's parents asked me to go on holiday with them?

- I overheard a group gossiping about me?

- My team came top of the league?

Feeling words

Jealous	Suspicious	Gloomy	
Silly	Awful	Sad	Puzzled
Unsure	Delighted	Furious	Happy
Satisfied	Tense	Weak	Loving
Anxious	Scared	Guilty	Depressed
Empty	Nervous	Bored	Confused
Grumpy	Embarrassed	Cheerful	

This list gives only a small number of words describing feelings. Try to find as many examples of your own as possible.

SECTION 1: PSYCHOLOGICAL ASPECTS OF HEALTH

ACTIVITY 9 — *The meaning of assertiveness*

Purpose To explore the differences between assertive, aggressive and passive behaviours

Time needed 30 minutes

What you need Sheets of paper. Pens. A copy of Activity Sheet 9 for each student.

How you do it

1. Explain that they are going to look at the variety of ways in which people can react in different situations. For example, ask them to imagine that they lend a book to someone in their class. When it's returned, there is writing all over the inside cover. Do they:
   - ignore it and say nothing
   - get angry and yell at the person who borrowed the book
   - say that they notice someone's written in it and ask if they know anything about it
   - respond in some other way?

2. Ask them to think of situations they've been in in which they weren't sure how to react. Make a list of these on the board. Alternatively you could come with different situations prepared on pieces of card.

3. Divide the class into groups of four. Give each group a different situation. They have 2 minutes to write down as many responses as they can to that situation. How might people respond? They are not to make any judgement at this stage about what it might be best to do.

4. Talk through Activity Sheet 9, pointing out the differences between assertive, aggressive and passive behaviours.

5. Check that they understand by asking each group to read out their situation and give an example from their list of an aggressive response. Ask them what the likely consequences would be and how the people on the receiving end would feel. What would happen if they acted in that way?

6. Repeat the process with passive and assertive responses.

Processing questions

- What is likely to happen if someone is aggressive/passive/assertive most of the time?
- Can the same words be assertive/aggressive/passive?
- What else makes a difference?
- What stops people from being assertive?

SECTION 1: PSYCHOLOGICAL ASPECTS OF HEALTH

Suggestions for follow-up work

In small groups, ask them to think of *one* of the following:

a situation where it would be OK to be passive
a situation where it would be OK to be aggressive
a situation where it would be OK to be assertive

Ask each group to make up a short play to show their situation to the rest of the class. The others guess what type of response it is and discuss its appropriateness.

SECTION 1: PSYCHOLOGICAL ASPECTS OF HEALTH

ACTIVITY SHEET 9
Differences between aggressive, passive and assertive behaviour

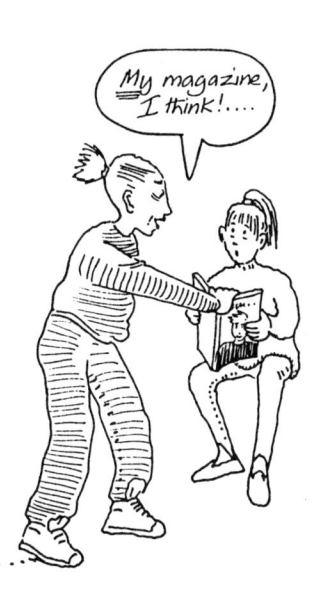

Aggressive

You do . . .

- try to get your own way, no matter what
- often leave other people feeling bad
- make yourself unpopular
- bully, fight, threaten, be sarcastic.

You don't . . .

- care how others feel
- respect the fact that they have rights too
- look for ways where you both end up feeling OK, possibly through a compromise.

Passive

You do . . .

- just hope that you'll get what you want
- rely on others to guess what you want or do things for you
- hide your real feelings and bottle things up
- sigh, sulk, hint, wish
- feel put upon.

You don't . . .

- ask for what you want
- stand up for yourself
- say how you feel
- feel good about yourself
- usually get what you want.

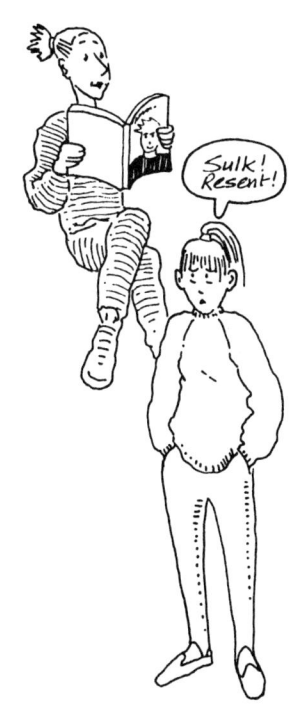

---

33 © A Picture of Health Permission to photocopy this page for participant use

Section 1: Psychological Aspects of Health

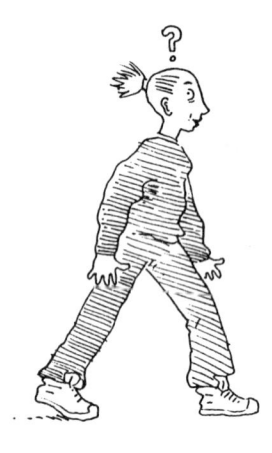

Assertive

You do . . .

- ask for what you want
- know you have rights
- listen to others and respect their rights
- say how you feel clearly
- believe in yourself.

You don't . . .

- think it's all about winning, no matter what
- expect others to guess what you want
- become over-anxious.

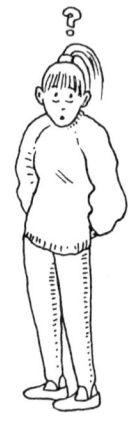

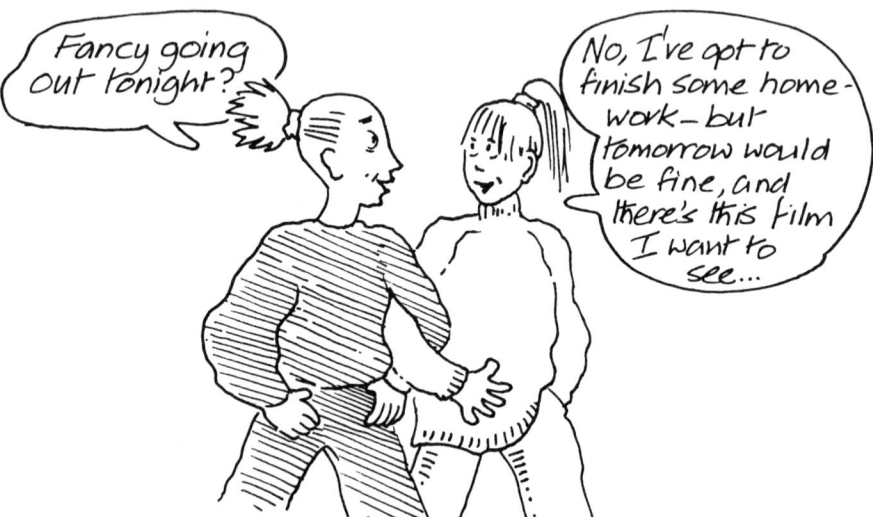

"Fancy going out tonight?"

"No, I've got to finish some homework – but tomorrow would be fine, and there's this film I want to see..."

SECTION 1: PSYCHOLOGICAL ASPECTS OF HEALTH

ACTIVITY 10 — *Being assertive*

Purpose To help students to practise being assertive

Time needed 30 minutes

What you need A copy of Activity Sheet 10A for each student. Prepared role cards as on Activity Sheet 10B.

How you do it
1. Read through Activity Sheet 10A with the students.
2. Explain that the more they practise being assertive, the easier it becomes. Ask them to work in groups of three, one person to be C, the observer, and the others to be A or B. Ask them to be aware of how they are sitting or standing, as this could have an effect on the conversation. C should be able to see what is happening but should not crowd the others or get in the way.
3. Give each group the same situation from Activity Sheet 10B. Allow time for them to read through their role card and to think about the situation and how they might feel. Don't let them get into discussion but encourage them to try it out.
4. After two or three minutes, stop them. Within each group, ask A and B to share how they felt. Did anything make them angry/upset/pleased? Ask C to feed back what s/he noticed.
5. Give each trio another situation from Activity Sheet 10B and repeat the process, with a different person playing the role of C. Then repeat for the final situation from Activity Sheet 10B, so each person takes the role of C once.
6. Bring the small groups together to discuss what they have learned.

Processing questions
- Was any situation more difficult than another? What made it so?
- Is it easier to be assertive with some people than with others?
- Did C notice anything which A or B had missed?
- Can they think of times when being assertive might not be the best thing?
- Can they think of other situations where it would be helpful to be assertive?

Suggestions for follow-up work Ask each student to think of one situation involving another person which they have experienced in which they would like to be more assertive. Get them to jot this down on card, describing briefly the other person involved. In their trios, they next take it in turn to read out their situation and explain to the others what the other person involved might feel like. Don't let them spend too long on this. Each person then takes it in turn to play themself, with the remaining two people in the trio taking the part of the other person or of C. After each role play, ask them to discuss how they felt, what seemed to be effective, what didn't work, what they could learn from this that might help in real life. This discussion should take at least as long as the role play itself.

SECTION 1: PSYCHOLOGICAL ASPECTS OF HEALTH

ACTIVITY SHEET 10A

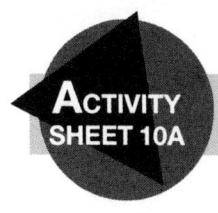

How to be assertive

Remember . . .

- being assertive doesn't mean getting your own way. Other people have rights too. You're aiming for a situation where everyone feels OK.
- to be assertive, you need to feel that you have a right to say how you feel and what you want. You need to value yourself and your rights.
- to be assertive you need to know what you want and how you feel and to be able to tell others clearly and directly. If you don't know or are unsure, how can you tell anyone else?
- it's not just what you say, but how you say it. Do you sound angry, accusing or unsure of yourself?
- you can give lots of clues about how you feel with your face and movements. Frowning can make you look cross or puzzled. Pointing your finger at someone can seem quite threatening. Looking away or at the floor can be off-putting to the person you're talking to. They may think you're not interested in them, or too shy to look at them. Folding your arms can make a barrier between you and the person you're talking to. There's a lot to think about!
- if you are assertive, you don't blame others by saying such things as 'You make me really angry' and 'You never help out.' Instead, start sentences with 'I' to show you're saying what *you* feel, not making a general comment about the other person. For example, 'I get angry when . . .' and 'I get really tired and fed up when I am left on my own to clear up.'
- if you would like something changed, be specific about what it is, and offer some ideas as to what would help.
- sometimes it may be better *not* to be assertive. It might not be worth it. Can you think of times when it might be better to keep quiet, times when it might be better to walk away, and times when it might be better to lose your temper? In each situation, you need to have some idea of what might happen if you behave in a certain way.
- what you want is to have a choice about how you behave . . . not always to react in the same way . . . but it can be difficult to break old habits. It takes practice!

© A Picture of Health   Permission to photocopy this page for participant use

SECTION 1: PSYCHOLOGICAL ASPECTS OF HEALTH

ACTIVITY SHEET 10B

How to be assertive

Photocopy and cut up before use.

--- ✂ ---

Situation 1

Person A B is a friend. S/he asks you home after school to see her/his new computer. There's nobody else in the house. Your friend sees a packet of cigarettes that her/his brother has left lying around, and takes two, saying 'Have one of these. He won't miss them.' You don't smoke and aren't keen. What will you say?

Person B You ask your friend, A, back home to see your new computer. There's nobody else in the house. You've been wanting to try a cigarette for a while now, although your mother would be very upset if she caught you smoking. She doesn't like the fact that your elder brother smokes. You see a packet of cigarettes which your brother has left lying around and take two. You'd like your friend to join you and say, 'Have one of these. He won't miss them.'

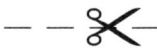

--- ✂ ---

Situation 2

Person A Someone in your class is having a party on Wednesday evening to which you're invited. You want to go as most of your friends will be there. It is likely to finish quite late and to go you would have to miss a regular commitment (eg football practice/piano lesson/gymnastics). Your parents do not usually let you go to parties during the week as you have school the next day. You decide to ask B, your mother/father.

Person B You are A's mother/father. You are worried that A doesn't take her/his schoolwork seriously and have therefore said that s/he is not allowed to go to any parties during the school week. Weekends are different, although you're not too happy about the crowd that A is hanging around with. Every Wednesday, A has a regular activity (eg football/piano/gymnastics) which you think is a good thing.

SECTION 1: PSYCHOLOGICAL ASPECTS OF HEALTH

---- ✂ ------------------------------

Situation 3

Person A At your local swimming pool, you go to buy a soft drink from a machine. You put in your money, but nothing happens. You find B, who works there, in order to ask how you can get your money back.

Person B You work at the local swimming pool. It has been a very busy morning. You've had a lot of trouble recently with teenagers trying to get money/drinks from the vending machines. A often comes to the pool. You've told her/him off a few times for messing about with her/his friends.

---- ✂ ------------------------------

Situations 1, 2 and 3

Person C You are the observer. Watch carefully to see:
- How A and B are sitting or standing. Do they lean forward/back/turn away/fidget?
- Whether they say clearly how they feel or what they want.
- Whether they listen to the other person, or interrupt/shout them down/ignore what s/he has said.

SECTION 1: PSYCHOLOGICAL ASPECTS OF HEALTH

ACTIVITY 11: *Positive strokes*

Purpose
- To encourage students to practise giving and receiving praise
- To encourage students to feel good about themselves

Time needed 30 minutes

What you need A group that knows one another well. Index cards. Pens.

How you do it
1. Write each student's name on two index cards.
2. Give out the cards face down, making sure that students do not receive their own card or two cards with the same name on them.
3. Explain that the purpose of the activity is to give a gift to someone, a positive message.
4. Ask them to write a message to the person named on each card, either 'If I were you, I'd feel good about a) ....; b) ....' or 'What I like about you is a) ....; b) ....'.
5. It is up to them whether they sign their message or leave it anonymous.
6. Collect in the cards and give each to the person named on it.
7. Divide the group into fours. Ask each person to share the comment about them which they like most.

Processing questions
- How does it feel to hear good things about themselves?
- Were they surprised by any of the comments made?
- Is that how they see themselves?
- How did they feel about this activity?
- Can they think of other ways of giving one another positive comments?

Suggestions for follow-up work Ask them to decide on someone to give a compliment, praise or encouragement to. It could be someone at home, someone else in the class, or someone who gives a good service. What are they going to say? Tell them to try it out, and get them to share their experiences at a later session.

SECTION 2

Environmental aspects of health

Section 2: Environmental Aspects of Health

Activity 12 — What is a healthy person?

Purpose
- To encourage students to explore ideas of what is meant by a 'healthy person'
- To encourage them to recognise that being healthy involves physical, mental and social health

Time needed 30 minutes

What you need A copy of Activity Sheet 12 for each student

How you do it
1. Ask each student to read each statement on Activity Sheet 12 and tick the six which they think are most important. They should do this as quickly as possible so they give their first reaction.
2. Get them to share their answers with a partner.
3. Bring the class together to compare results and share their ideas about health. Draw out the physical, mental and social aspects of health.

Processing questions
- In their six statements, did they have a balance of mental, social and physical health?
- In sharing with someone else, did they have similar or different views of being healthy?
- Is being healthy different from not being ill?
- Is it to do with feeling good in your mind as well as your body?
- Is being healthy about living to a great age?
- Do some people only think of being healthy as something to do with how they look?
- How much is our health affected by the environment in which we live?

Suggestions for follow-up work
- Ask students to interview three people of different ages to find out what sort of person they think of as a healthy person. Get them to bring the results to the class to compare people's views on what makes a healthy person.
- Collect pictures and references to health in newspapers and magazines. They can be used in Activity 18.

SECTION 2: ENVIRONMENTAL ASPECTS OF HEALTH

ACTIVITY SHEET 12

What is a healthy person?

Read through the following list and tick six statements which you think are the most important qualities needed by a person in order for them to be regarded as healthy.

A healthy person . . .

- [ ] 1 Is never ill
- [ ] 2 Can run for a bus without getting out of breath
- [ ] 3 Takes life easily without getting upset
- [ ] 4 Makes friends easily
- [ ] 5 Has access to good health services
- [ ] 6 Has a comfortable home
- [ ] 7 Takes regular exercise
- [ ] 8 Is anyone who has reached 75 years of age
- [ ] 9 Avoids smoking and drugs which damage health
- [ ] 10 Lives in a clean environment
- [ ] 11 Is able to cope with any disability s/he has (eg deafness or being confined to a wheelchair)
- [ ] 12 Is able to make the best of the situation s/he is in
- [ ] 13 Feels well all the time
- [ ] 14 Avoids foods with chemicals in them
- [ ] 15 Never seems depressed
- [ ] 16 Has a good figure
- [ ] 17 Doesn't take pills and medicines
- [ ] 18 Is careful about personal hygiene
- [ ] 19 Takes care to have all the right injections (immunisation)
- [ ] 20 Feels good about her/himself
- [ ] 21 Has a belief which helps her/him through life
- [ ] 22 Eats regular meals rather than snacks
- [ ] 23 Hardly ever visits the doctor
- [ ] 24 Has clear skin

© A Picture of Health   Permission to photocopy this page for participant use

SECTION 2: ENVIRONMENTAL ASPECTS OF HEALTH

ACTIVITY 13 — Influences on health

Purpose
- To identify the positive and negative influences on health
- To demonstrate that health may be affected by a person's behaviour, but health problems are also created by social and environmental factors

Time 30 minutes

What you need Copies of the scenarios on Activity Sheet 13. A flipchart, board or OHP. Pens. Paper.

How you do it
1. Ask the students to work in groups of three or four.
2. Give each group a card with a scenario to read. Ask them to list all the things which they think are influencing the person concerned.
3. Once they have done that, they should answer the questions at the bottom of the card.
4. Back in the whole group, ask them to draw up a list of all the influences identified. Write these up so all can see them.

Processing questions
- In their small groups, did they think of anything positive that could be done to improve people's health?
- What actions can people take to protect their own health?
- How much is it their responsibility?
- Are there influences on our health which we can't control?
- Are there health problems related to particular jobs?
- What safety and protective measures could help?
- Can groups, organisations or the government do anything to help?

Suggestions for follow-up work Ask students to write their own scenario which illustrates influences on health, for example:

work environment
housing
peer pressure
advertising
pollution
self-image

SECTION 2: ENVIRONMENTAL ASPECTS OF HEALTH

Scenarios

ACTIVITY SHEET 13

Photocopy and cut up before use.

---- ✂ ----------------------------

.... **Selina** ....

. . . is a shift worker in a small textile factory making dresses/ clothing. Her job is cutting out thick layers of material. This is done with an electrically operated band-saw. It is often easier to work the machine without the safety guard. Meal breaks are taken in a grubby room and most of the workers bring their own food. The toilets lead off this room.

Questions
- What effect do you think conditions in the factory have on Selina's health?
- What do you think the employer should do?
- Are there things Selina herself can do?
- Who else might be involved?
- What questions would you want to ask if you were going to start work in a factory or large organisation?

---- ✂ ----------------------------

.... **Rachel** ....

. . . has just started work. She was interviewed and given tests to find out what she would be best at doing. She took part in the company's training before starting work on the shop floor. There is a staff canteen but she prefers to get out at lunchtime and often meets her friends in the local pub. She has twice been late back and has obviously been drinking alcohol. She enjoys using the company's sports facilities. The medical services offer all employees regular health check-ups.

Questions
- What effect do you think her working conditions have on Rachel's health?
- What are the important things that her employer has done for Rachel and her fellow-workers?
- Could anything else be done?
- Are there things that Rachel can do to improve her health?
- What questions would you want to ask if you were going to start work in a factory or large organisation?

SECTION 2: ENVIRONMENTAL ASPECTS OF HEALTH

Paul

... is 13. He suffers from diabetes. This means he has to take regular doses of insulin to keep up his blood sugar level. If he forgets, he can look pale, feel faint and dizzy, and have a lot of sweating. On one occasion he lost consciousness.

Questions
- How can Paul's classmates help him with his diabetes?
- Can the school or teachers help in any way?
- What are the things that Paul can do to keep himself as healthy as possible?
- Can you think of other conditions which affect people's health over a long period of time?
- Is there any group or organisation that can do anything to help?

---------- ✂ ----------

Steve

... travels home by train during the rush hour. It is often impossible to get in the non-smoking end of the compartment. A crowd of lads regularly light up as soon as they're on the train. This upsets a lot of the passengers.

Questions
- Can the smoke from other people's cigarettes harm you?
- What action can Steve take in this situation?
- In any situation, should the rights of a non-smoker come before the rights of a smoker? Why or why not?
- Could more be done by the government, industry and other organisations to restrict smoking in public places?

---------- ✂ ----------

Melanie

... is 13 and does a paper round every weekday, to earn pocket money to go on a skiing trip with her friends. She gets up before 6 every morning and has now been asked to work on Sundays as well. She has a busy social life and is finding it difficult to fit her schoolwork in with everything else.

Questions
- What effect do you think her present job has on Melanie's health?
- What do you think her employer should do to make sure she's not coming to any harm?
- Are there things Melanie herself can do?
- Who else might be concerned?
- What questions would you want to ask if you were offered a part-time job?

© A Picture of Health   Permission to photocopy this page for participant use

SECTION 2: ENVIRONMENTAL ASPECTS OF HEALTH

ACTIVITY 14
Infectious/non-infectious diseases

Purpose
- To enable students to distinguish between infectious and non-infectious diseases.

Time needed 30 minutes

What you need A copy of Activity Sheet 14A and 14B for each student. Pens.

How you do it
1. Give each student a copy of Activity Sheet 14A
2. Ask them to ring round those diseases they think are infectious (contagious).
3. Ask them to underline those that can be prevented by immunisation.
4. Ask them to write down the names of those which might be caused by a person's lifestyle/behaviour.
5. Bring the class together to discuss the different causes of ill-health.

Processing questions
- Are there some diseases that are more difficult to control and do something about than others (eg hereditary diseases)?
- Are there some that may be due to the environment in which people live (eg illness due to dirty drinking water)?
- Are there some that are more associated with old age (eg arthritis)?
- Do they know the ages at which immunisations are given? Activity Sheet 14B gives some information to be used as appropriate.

Suggestions for follow-up work
- Get students to find out how patterns of ill-health have changed in the last hundred years, and write an account of the reasons for the changes.
- Ask them to collect information about immunisation from a local health promotion unit or surgery. Get them to prepare a statement about any leaflets or posters, saying whether they find them clear, attractive and easy to read. Ask if the documents tell people what they need to know.

SECTION 2: ENVIRONMENTAL ASPECTS OF HEALTH

ACTIVITY SHEET 14A

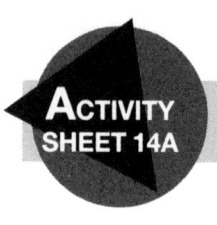

Spot the difference

Flu	German measles
Verruca	Herpes simplex (cold sores)
Poliomyelitis	Bronchitis
Chicken pox	Tuberculosis
Lung cancer	Whooping cough
Acne	Food poisoning
Diabetes	HIV
Broken leg	Eczema
Asthma	Common cold
Coronary heart disease	Measles

Put a ring round those which you think are infectious.
Underline, in colour, those that can be prevented by immunisation.

SECTION 2: ENVIRONMENTAL ASPECTS OF HEALTH

ACTIVITY SHEET 14B

Immunisation facts

At 2 months, 3 months and 4 months	Diphtheria, tetanus and whooping cough (DTP)	One combined injection each month
	Polio	By mouth each month
At 12–18 months (usually before 15 months)	Measles, mumps, rubella (MMR)	One combined injection
By 5 years (around school entry)	Diphtheria, tetanus	One combined injection
	Polio	By mouth

Do you know what immunisations you have had?

Why is it important for girls to have a second immunisation against rubella at 15 years?

Do you know that you should have a tetanus booster every ten years?

Do you know that it is important to check what immunisations you need before visiting countries outside Europe?

© A Picture of Health   Permission to photocopy this page for participant use

SECTION 2: ENVIRONMENTAL ASPECTS OF HEALTH

ACTIVITY 15 — *Card sort*

Purpose
- To help students understand the causes of infectious diseases, how they are spread and how they can be prevented

Time needed 30 minutes

What you need A copy of Activity Sheet 15A for each student. Sets of cards (see Activity Sheet 15B) for each group – disease, how it spreads, and how it is controlled.

How you do it
1. Point out that most infectious diseases are caused by bacteria and viruses, commonly called germs. Give each student Activity Sheet 15A to look at.
2. Working in threes or fours, give each group a complete set of cards (see Activity Sheet 15B). Ask them to lay out the cards with the heading **Disease** on the left-hand side of their desk in a column.
3. Now get them to take the **How it spreads** cards. Each of these fits alongside one of the **Disease** cards. See if they can fit the correct method of spread to each disease. In some cases the methods of spread will be the same.
4. Do the same with the **How it is controlled** cards.
5. Tell each group to change places with another group, to compare results.
6. Talk students through the answer sheet (the original of Activity Sheet 15B) and encourage discussion about the ways in which diseases are spread.

Processing questions
- What are the ways in which individuals can prevent the spread of infection?
- In what kind of places are you most likely to pick up infections?
- Why is it dangerous to swim in water where there is a sewage outfall?
- Why are people more vulnerable to infection after an operation?
- Why are there strict regulations for bringing dogs into the country?
- Are some bacteria useful?

Suggestions for follow-up work Ask them to find out all they can about one of the following people:
Joseph Lister
Robert Jenner
Louis Pasteur
Alexander Fleming.

SECTION 2: ENVIRONMENTAL ASPECTS OF HEALTH

ACTIVITY SHEET 15A

Card sort

.... **Bacteria** ....

– are very small – one million would cover a pinhead
– live outside body cells wherever it is warm and moist and there is food
– often produce harmful substances called TOXINS (poisons)
– are usually killed by ANTIBIOTICS (some develop a resistance to antibiotics)
– cause the following diseases:
  boils
  food poisoning
  impetigo
  pneumonia
  sore throats
  tetanus
  typhoid

.... **Viruses** ....

– are only visible under an electron microscope – one million would fit inside a bacterium
– live inside body cells, where they bring about changes
– remain unharmed by antibiotics and so are difficult to treat
– cause the following diseases:
  colds
  chicken pox
  flu
  herpes
  measles
  mumps
  polio
  rubella
– in the 1980s a new virus was identified now called human immuno deficiency virus, or HIV. This is the virus which is believed to cause AIDS.

SECTION 2: ENVIRONMENTAL ASPECTS OF HEALTH

ACTIVITY SHEET 15B
Card sort

Cards

Photocopy this sheet and cut it into cards. The original serves as an answer sheet.

Disease TUBERCULOSIS	**How it spreads** Coughing. Damp living conditions	**How it is controlled** Vaccination and improved living conditions
Disease COMMON COLD	**How it spreads** Coughing and sneezing	**How it is controlled** Difficult
Disease INFLUENZA	**How it spreads** Coughing and sneezing	**How it is controlled** Difficult. Some vaccines have limited success
Disease DIPHTHERIA	**How it spreads** Dust	**How it is controlled** Vaccination
Disease IMPETIGO	**How it spreads** Touching. Contact with personal effects	**How it is controlled** Personal hygiene. Antibiotics. Antiseptic. Isolation
Disease ATHLETE'S FOOT	**How it spreads** Contact between feet and changing-room floors	**How it is controlled** Use footbaths in swimming pools. Good personal hygiene and careful drying of feet

© A Picture of Health   Permission to photocopy this page for participant use

SECTION 2: ENVIRONMENTAL ASPECTS OF HEALTH

Disease	How it spreads	How it is controlled
TYPHOID	Sewage in food and drinking water	Sewage treatment. Clean water supplies. Personal hygiene
MALARIA	Mosquito is carrier of the malarial parasite	Anti-malaria tablets. Draining land. Insecticides. Mosquito nets
RABIES	Bite from infected dog	Quarantine. Destruction of diseased animals. Vaccination
HEPATITIS B	Blood or objects in contact with blood, for example the use of a dirty needle for injection	High level of hygiene in hospitals and doctors' surgeries. Vaccination
HIV	Unprotected sexual intercourse. Injecting drug users sharing needles. Infected mother to unborn child.	Use of condoms. Blood screening. Needle exchange schemes. Health education
POLIO	Sewage in food and drinking water	Isolation. Closure of swimming pools. Good sanitation. Vaccination

SECTION 2: ENVIRONMENTAL ASPECTS OF HEALTH

Disease	**How it spreads**	**How it is controlled**
GERMAN MEASLES (RUBELLA)	Exhaled air	Vaccination

Disease	**How it spreads**	**How it is controlled**
SYPHILIS	Sexual intercourse	Antibiotics. Use of condoms. Health education

Disease	**How it spreads**	**How it is controlled**
GONORRHOEA	Sexual intercourse	Antibiotics. Use of condoms. Health education

SECTION 2: ENVIRONMENTAL ASPECTS OF HEALTH

ACTIVITY 16

Where to go for help

Purpose
- To inform students of the range of services and help available to them

Time 35–40 minutes

What you need A set of problem and solution cards (see Activity Sheet 16), one card for each person

How you do it
1. Give each student a card.
2. Explain that half the cards outline a problem and the other half have on them a person or an organisation that may be able to help solve a problem.
3. Ask students to move around the room trying to find a card that matches their own. Encourage them to discuss with one another what would be the best source of help.
4. Bring the class together to discuss any pairs of problems and sources of help they are not sure about.
5. Invite the class to compile a directory of useful contacts and sources of help.

Processing questions
- What are the qualities that are important in the person from whom you would seek help?
- Did they find it easy to agree on the source of help?
- Who are the other people who help with problems?

Suggestions for follow-up work
- Invite one of the professional helpers mentioned on the cards to come to talk about their work. The class can prepare questions they would like to ask about the work in advance.
- Students can collect problem pages concerned with health from teenage magazines. They can discuss the solutions offered and see if they agree with them. They can also look at what they have interpreted as health problems. Have they tended to define those narrowly?

SECTION 2: ENVIRONMENTAL ASPECTS OF HEALTH

ACTIVITY SHEET 16

Problem and solution cards

Photocopy onto card and cut up before use

Problem	**Source of help**
Jane is recovering from an accident and needs advice on appropriate exercises.	PHYSIOTHERAPIST
Pete is worried that his cold sores are contagious and can easily be passed on.	GP
Jaktar has an ear infection that won't clear up. He is a keen swimmer and thinks his hearing is being affected.	GP
Helen is upset because her Mum's boyfriend keeps coming into her room without asking and cuddling her when she doesn't want it.	TEACHER HELPLINE
Tim has had a lot of headaches recently and has difficulty reading small print.	OPTICIAN trained to test eyes as well as to supply glasses on prescription
Dave has a swollen toe where he cut the nail; he can hardly get his shoe on.	CHIROPODIST

SECTION 2: ENVIRONMENTAL ASPECTS OF HEALTH

Kelly has done some shoplifting recently. She is worried about what she has done and can't sleep at nights.	PARENT FRIEND TEACHER
Damien wants to take a job stacking supermarket shelves. He needs the cash but is doubtful if his school will provide the form he needs to get taken on.	TEACHER
Chris has crooked teeth and has been told that they will have to be straightened at some time. He is worried about this and how it will be done.	DENTIST
Kim knows that she must soon have BCG/rubella injections. She is terrified of needles.	SCHOOL NURSE GP
Rachel fell off her bike and may have broken her arm.	CASUALTY DEPARTMENT
Mandy thinks her older brother is taking drugs but is frightened to talk to him about it.	HELPLINE TEACHER PARENT PERSON CONCERNED

SECTION 2: ENVIRONMENTAL ASPECTS OF HEALTH

ACTIVITY 17 — A visit to the doctor

Purpose To identify and practise the skills students need when they visit the doctor

Time needed 45 minutes

What you need Flipchart or OHT. Copies of case-studies on Activity Sheet 17 for each group. Felt tip pens.

How you do it

1. In pairs, ask them to find out if they know:
   - the name and address of their doctor
   - whether the surgery has an appointments system
   - how to contact the doctor or what to do in an emergency
   - if there are other professionals who work at the surgery (eg practice nurse).

2. Invite students to think about a visit they have made to their doctor and to share their feelings about the visit. Prompts could be: annoyance at being kept waiting; anxiety about what was going to happen; feeling awkward or shy at asking questions. Emphasise that the sharing is about their feelings and not about their illness.

3. Record the range of feelings on a flipchart.

4. Ask students to think of ways in which visits could be made easier or more comfortable. Record the strategies that are suggested. Does it help to have a parent or friend with them?

5. Divide the class into groups of four. Give each group a copy of Activity Sheet 17. Each group should choose a case-study that interests them and answer the following questions:
   - What would the person in the case-study expect from the doctor?
   - What would the person need to tell the doctor?
   - What questions would the person need to ask?
   - What questions might the doctor ask?

6. Bring the group together to discuss how to get the most from a visit to the doctor. What skills are involved?

Processing questions
- How can they prepare for the visit? (eg by writing down any symptoms or questions they want to ask beforehand)
- What can they do to help themselves to be more confident in explaining symptoms to a doctor?
- How can they be clear about what they need to ask?
- What are the skills they need when they are at the surgery? (eg being able to speak clearly about what is really worrying them, looking at

Section 2: Environmental Aspects of Health

the doctor as they speak, checking that they have understood any advice or instructions from the doctor before they leave)
- Are doctors allowed to divulge information about their patients?

Sugestions for follow-up work
- Get them to find out what they have to do to register with a doctor.
- Tell them to ask relations and friends what kind of things they think help patient/doctor relationships. List their suggestions.

SECTION 2: ENVIRONMENTAL ASPECTS OF HEALTH

ACTIVITY SHEET 17

A visit to the doctor – case-studies

Each of the following young people has decided to visit her/his doctor. Read through the case-studies and decide which one to work on.

Chris

. . . is going on a hitch-hiking trip to Spain. He gets an allergic reaction from insect stings. He swells up quickly where the bite occurs and feels dizzy. He is worried and unsure about what he can do to protect himself.

Selina

. . . is a keen athlete. She has been training for over a year. It is two days before a big race and she has severe pain in the muscles of her lower leg. She went on with her training until her legs became so painful that she had to see the doctor.

Angie

. . . feels off-colour. She works hard at school but is finding things more and more of a struggle. She feels depressed and her best friend has just left to live in another part of the country.

Ted

. . . has decided he wants to become a vegetarian. He is small for his age and his mother is worried about him eating a proper diet.

Bob

. . . started to have severe headaches. He had a bad knock on his head some months ago and is worried that the headaches might have something to do with this.

SECTION 2: ENVIRONMENTAL ASPECTS OF HEALTH

ACTIVITY 18
The influence of the media and advertising

Purpose
- To help students understand the impact of the media and advertising on attitudes towards health
- To help them understand how advertisers use a range of techniques to promote their products

Time 30 minutes

What you need Newspapers. Magazines. Scissors. Glue. Felt-tip pens. A copy of Activity Sheet 18 for each student. Sheets of paper labelled as shown in Section 2 below.

How you do it
1. Divide the class into groups and give each a pile of newspapers and magazines. Ask them to cut out any advertisements carrying health messages.
2. Give each group four large sheets of paper labelled:
   i   These can damage your health
   ii These claim to contribute to health
   iii These promote health and give information about health
   iv These are neutral, leaving you to make up your own mind.
   Tell each group to sort their advertisements and stick them on the appropriate sheet.
3. Give each group copies of Activity Sheet 18 to help them analyse the ways in which advertisers promote their message or product.
4. Bring the groups together to share their views about the way health messages are promoted.

Processing questions
- Which category had the most advertisements? Why do they think this is? Who pays for the advertisement?
- Which advertisements do they like best? Why?
- How were these advertisements persuasive? Was it the size? The use of colour? The use of famous names to endorse products? The use of competitions with valuable prizes?
- Can we get conflicting health messages from the same source?
- How can we assess the truth of the health messages?
- Who has the most money to spend on advertisements?
- What effect do advertising hoardings have on the environment?

Suggestions for follow-up work
- Suggest they carry out a survey among their families and friends to discover their favourite advertisements on TV. What makes them appealing? Does it encourage them to buy the products or take the advice offered?

Section 2: Environmental Aspects of Health

- Over 1.25 million magazines are sold to teenagers each week. Ask students to make a detailed study of one issue of a magazine to see how much space is devoted to particular features (eg fashion, romance, pop, sport, hobbies, problems, advertisements). Are there differences between boys' and girls' magazines? What views do they think the editors have of young people?

SECTION 2: ENVIRONMENTAL ASPECTS OF HEALTH

ACTIVITY SHEET 18

Decoding sheet

Place a tick to show which techniques were used in your advertisements.

	Adverts which can damage your health	Adverts making health claims	Adverts for health promotion
EXAMPLE	Cigarette	'Clears the skin'	'Don't drink and drive'
Techniques			
Use of sex appeal			
Wealth			
Humour			
Strength/macho appeal			
Use of a famous name, personality			
Competitions			
Giving factual information			
Attractiveness of people involved			
Any other techniques?			

SECTION 2: ENVIRONMENTAL ASPECTS OF HEALTH

ACTIVITY 19 — *Attitudes to the environment*

Purpose	• To explore different attitudes to the environment
Time needed	30 minutes
What you need	Flipchart or board. A copy of Activity Sheet 19 for each student. Pens.
How you do it	1 Ask students to think about a place they enjoy going to or being in.
	2 Invite them, in pairs, to describe to each other these special places and the reason for their choice.
	3 Bring the class together to discuss what makes an environment 'special'. Record the suggestions on the flipchart or board.
	4 Repeat the exercise, asking them to think about what makes an environment hostile.
	5 Give each person a copy of Activity Sheet 19 to complete.
	6 Invite them to share their answers with a partner.
Processing questions	• Which statements did they have different answers to in their pairs?
	• Are there things we can do to improve a hostile environment?
	• Do people share the same views about their environment?
	• Do our views change according to what is going on at the time?
	• Whose responsibility is it to bring about improvements in the environment? Is it individuals? Local councils? Government?
	• Can students think of particular examples where improvements have been achieved? Who was responsible?
Suggestions for follow-up work	• They could use Activity Sheet 19 with other people (eg family and friends) to find out their views on the environment. Are there differences between younger and older people?
	• Get them to find out the names of organisations that set out to campaign for the environment, and to make a collection of their literature. Ask how they would choose which ones to support.
	• Organise a project for the class in which they set out to improve an aspect of their own environment of their choice.

SECTION 2: ENVIRONMENTAL ASPECTS OF HEALTH

ACTIVITY SHEET 19

Attitudes to the environment

Different people hold different views about the environment. Below are some comments made by people about the environment. Do you agree with them? Tick each as quickly as possible.

	Agree	Don't know	Disagree
'Most beaches are too filthy for swimming'			
'Playing loud music in public should be forbidden'			
'Acid rain has nothing to do with us'			
'Smoking should be banned in public places'			
'Everyone is responsible in some way for pollution'			
'Posters and advertisements on hoardings spoil the environment'			
'We need more green areas and play areas, not supermarkets'			
'It's easier to put things in the dustbin than sort them for recycling'			
'The car does more harm to the environment than anything else'			

© A Picture of Health   Permission to photocopy this page for participant use

SECTION 2: ENVIRONMENTAL ASPECTS OF HEALTH

ACTIVITY 20: *A healthy community*

Purpose
- To share their ideas about what makes a healthy community
- To learn more about their own community provision for health

Time needed 25 minutes and follow-up

What you need Large-scale street map(s) of the local area. Coloured stickers or pins. Plain cards. Coloured string. Flipchart or OHT. Pens. Paper.

How you do it
1. Working in small groups, students draw up a list of what they would expect to find in a 'healthy' community.
2. Each group feeds back the results to draw up a composite class list on a flipchart or OHT. Check to see whether they have included:
   - health care facilities (eg hospitals, clinics, health centres)
   - education facilities (eg schools, colleges, community centres)
   - facilities for the elderly, handicapped (eg day centres, rest homes)
   - childcare facilities (eg clinics, nurseries, playgrounds)
   - help/information agencies (eg Citizens' Advice Bureaux, Samaritans)
   - adequate housing
   - good street lighting
   - shopping areas with facilities for young mothers and children and easy access for the disabled
   - pedestrian precincts.
3. Print each suggestion about facilities/amenities on a small plain card.

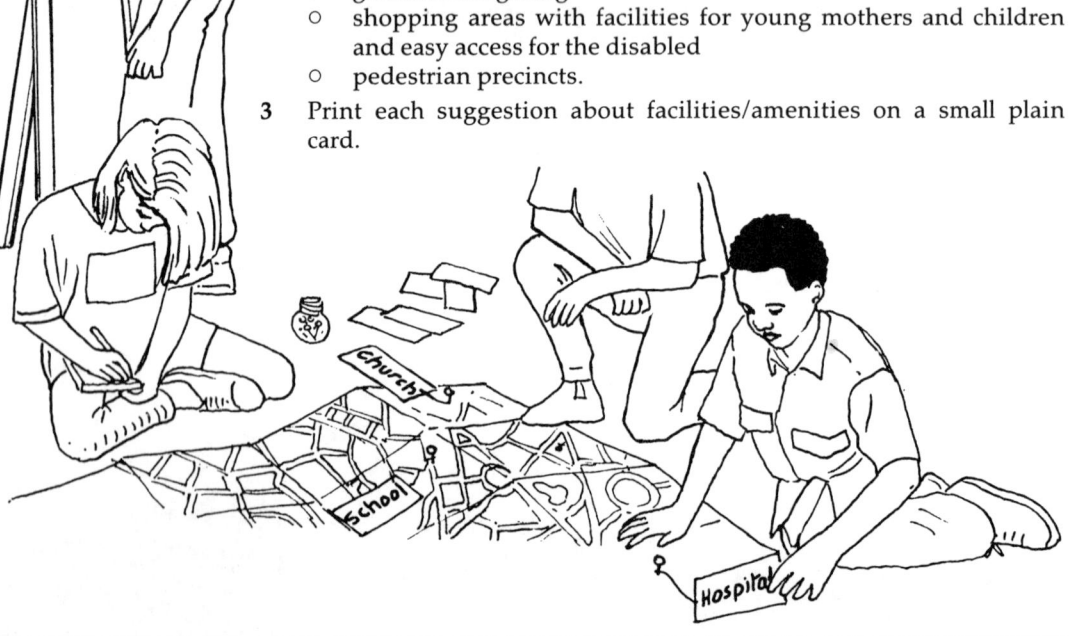

Section 2: Environmental Aspects of Health

4   Divide the area map(s) into sectors, allocating one sector to each group. Using stickers or pins, show on the map the facilities, agencies, clinics etc which were written on the cards.

5   Link the stickers/pins to the cards with coloured string, and display the map.

Processing questions
- What does the finished map tell them about their community?
- Could they locate all the suggestions made for their community? If not, why was this?
- What are the things which contribute to an unhealthy community? Prompts might include: derelict areas, ill-lit streets, dangerous footpaths, poor refuse collection, factories producing toxic waste.
- To what extent do good facilities make a community healthy?
- What else is needed? Point out that the people living in an area are a great resource. To be effective they need to know what services are available and how to use them, to understand what they need to be healthy, to feel cared for and to care about the health of everyone else.

Suggestions for follow-up work
- Ask students to carry out more detailed surveys of one of the aspects on the cards.
- Get them to find out more about the 'Healthy Cities' Project.
- Get them to find out about all the people in the community with special health knowledge (eg health visitor, chemist, chiropodist, acupuncturist). Where can they be found? What type of information/help can they give?

SECTION 3

Sex education

Section 3: Sex Education

Activity 21: Me as a member of a group

Purpose
- To identify the range of groups to which students belong
- To explore the benefits and disadvantages of being in a group

Time needed 30 minutes

What you need Large sheets of paper. Coloured felt-tip pens.

How you do it

1. Ask the students, working with four or five others, to brainstorm the types of groups that they belonged to when they were 8 or 9. Ask them to think about groups at school and at home (eg friends, family, class at school, football club). With a different coloured pen, they should then underline any to which they still belong and discuss whether these groups have changed in any ways. Can they add any new groups to the list which apply now but did not when they were 8 or 9?

2. In the whole class, discuss any changes which they have identified in the types of groups to which they belong. Do they feel differently about being a member of any of the groups? Which groups did they *choose* to belong to?

3. Divide the class into pairs and get each pair to select one type of group to which both chose to belong. What were their reasons for wanting to be in that group? Tell them to divide a sheet of paper in half, marking one side + and the other −. On it they should list any positive or good things about being in that group, and any negative or bad things. It may help them to think about times when they felt good or bad . . . what was happening?

Processing questions
- What are some of the good things that can come from being a member of a group?
- What are some of the bad?
- What sort of groups do they see themselves being part of in future?
- How important is it to fit in with the group?
- Are there any times when they think it would be important to do what they want or think is right, even though this might upset some of the group?

Suggestions for follow-up work

Ask them to write an essay on: 'A group I belong to. What it means to be a member.' Tell them to consider whether there are certain codes of behaviour, things which are expected of them or particular clothes which they have to wear.

Section 3: Sex Education

Activity 22: Friends

Purpose
- To identify and rank in order of importance the qualities students look for in a friend

Time needed 30–40 minutes

What you need Index cards, or a set of nine diamond-shaped cards for each student. Paper and pens.

How you do it
1. Ask students to think about someone whom they consider to be a friend. How do they know s/he is a friend? Each person writes down five words which they think describe a friend.
2. Ask them to share in groups of four what they have written and to agree on nine words. Give each student nine blank index cards or diamond-shaped cards. Ask them to write each of the nine words from their group on a different card. Working on their own, they then arrange them in order of importance in the shape of a diamond, putting the one which they think most important at the top, and the least important at the bottom.
3. With one person from their group, they now compare their diamond patterns and try to reach agreement. Then they join with the other two members of their group and again see if they can agree, at least on the top and bottom of the diamond.
4. Ask each group to appoint a spokesperson to feed back:
   - their lowest priority
   - how easy it was to agree.

Processing questions
- Did the groups come up with similar qualities which they would look for in friends?
- Were there any differences?
- Do boys look for different things in a friend than girls?
- Do they look for different qualities in friends of the same sex from those in friends of the opposite sex?

Suggestions for follow-up-work
Ask the students to interview an older family member about a friend who was important to them when they were in their early teens. What were they looking for in a friend? Are the same things important in the friends they have today?

Section 3: Sex Education

Activity 23: Listening skills

Purpose
- To help students understand the importance of active listening
- To practise active listening

Time needed 30 minutes

What you need Flipchart paper and pens

How you do it

1. Explain that one quality that we often need from a friend is a willingness to listen to us, to be there for us. Paying full attention to someone is a skill which we can develop.
2. Each student chooses a partner and the pairs decide who will be A and who will be B. A is to speak for 2 minutes about a holiday that s/he has had. B makes it obvious that s/he isn't listening by not looking at A, saying nothing, yawning and so on.
3. After time is up, get A and B to tell one another how it felt to talk without being listened to and to avoid listening. Did they find it easy to keep going?
4. Next, ask B in each group to talk for 2 minutes about a friend who was important to her/him when s/he was younger. A is to listen, showing that s/he is involved, but not interrupting or speaking.
5. Talk for a few minutes about how easy it was to speak/to keep talking.
6. Finally, ask A to talk for 2 minutes about a time when s/he was helped by a friend. B is to listen, showing s/he is listening in the way that seems appropriate – talking if that encourages A to speak.
7. Ask A and B to talk again about how it felt, comparing the three conversations. They should say how easy it was to talk and to listen. Ask them to think about how they can tell if someone is listening or not, and about what makes it difficult to listen.
8. Ask each pair to join with two other pairs to make a group of six. Together they draw up a list of how they knew that someone was listening – thinking about what they did and said.
9. As a whole class, compare the lists that have been drawn up.

Processing questions
- How easy is it to tell if someone is listening?
- How do they show they are listening?
- Have people considered body posture/eye contact/facial expression?

Suggestions for follow-up work Activity 24 offers a further opportunity to practise listening.

SECTION 3: SEX EDUCATION

ACTIVITY 24 — *Where do I stand?*

Purpose
- To encourage students to explore attitudes to relationships and sexuality
- To listen to the opinions of others
- To be aware of the range of sexual attitudes in society
- To experience movement in the session

Time needed 30 minutes

What you need A large clear space. Four large sheets of paper, each with one of the following on it: STRONGLY AGREE, AGREE WITH RESERVATIONS, DISAGREE WITH RESERVATIONS, STRONGLY DISAGREE. Several statements likely to generate a range of opinions. (Choose from the statements below or write your own, appropriate to the group. Once students are used to the process, encourage them to come up with statements of their own.)

How you do it
1. Explain that this activity offers them a chance to work out where they stand on certain issues and to practise listening to others. Stress that the stand anyone takes is not fixed in concrete. They may change their minds tomorrow, or even during the activity.
2. Place the sheets of paper in a continuum along the floor with plenty of space between them.
3. Read out a statement and ask students to move to a place on the continuum which best fits their opinion on the statement. Start with statements which are non-threatening and gradually move to more controversial ones. Students have the right to abstain from expressing their opinion on any statement.
4. When everyone has taken a stand, ask them to turn to someone near them and discuss the reasons why they are there. Encourage them to listen to one another; someone else may be there for a very different reason from their own.
5. After a couple of minutes, tell them to find someone standing at a different point and repeat the process.
6. Repeat the whole process with two or three more statements.

Processing questions
- How did they feel doing that activity, that is taking a stand?
- How do they think it felt if someone found her/himself on her/his own at a point on the continuum?
- Which issues did they find easy/difficult?
- Did they want to change their position after listening to someone else?
- Was it easy for them to listen to someone who had a different opinion?

Section 3: Sex Education

Possible statements   A good friend is someone who will tell me the truth
It is natural for women to be more caring than men
It is not OK for a girl to ask a boy out
Twelve-year-old girls are always more grown up than boys
Young people these days are more careful about whom they sleep with
It is embarrassing for a girl to carry a condom
Boys are more interested in sex than girls
There is nothing wrong with feeling attracted to someone of the same sex
Contraception is the responsibility of both partners who have decided to have sex
The age of sexual consent should be lowered
The best way of avoiding HIV infection is to use a condom

SECTION 3: SEX EDUCATION

ACTIVITY 25 — *Different values*

Purpose
- To discuss moral values
- To explore those held by different cultures and groups

Time needed 30–45 minutes

What you need Various duplicated pieces of stimulus materials – either articles/stories written by people from various cultures, or short programmes such as 'Asian Girl' in the BBC Schools Topics series. Examples of written materials are given in Activity Sheet 25.

How you do it

1. Point out that people hold different attitudes about sexuality, in particular about what is right and wrong. Ask students where they think these attitudes come from. Stress that their religious beliefs and the culture in which they were brought up will affect their attitudes. Some people are influenced by two cultures. For example, a Sikh girl may lead one life at home (with Indian clothes, food and Punjabi language) and another at school (with a uniform, English language and English food).

2. In order to avoid crude stereotyping, use materials describing the experiences of real people. Either show them a video such as 'Asian Girl', or divide the class into pairs giving each pair two or three pieces of stimulus material such as in Activity Sheet 25.

3. Ask them to discuss the messages which the people concerned seemed to be getting:
   - about the way they should look and behave
   - about relationships
   - about marriage and having children.

   Who are these messages from? Do any of them conflict? What sort of messages do students get from their own families? Do they agree with them all?

4. Encourage discussion in the whole group.

Processing questions
- What kinds of messages do people get from their family?
- Are girls likely to get different messages from boys?
- What are the advantages/disadvantages of living in a family with strong beliefs?
- Why is it important to recognise that some people have different beliefs from their own?

Suggestions for follow-up work Section 4 on family life education contains several activities which encourage discussion on different family lifestyles. Students may be interested in talking to representatives from various religious/cultural groups. Activity 39 describes the process of inviting visitors into school.

SECTION 3: SEX EDUCATION

Different values

ACTIVITY SHEET 25

DESTINE

Destine's family are Turkish Cypriot, from Northern Cyprus, where many of the family still live.

My father won't allow us to go out with boys although the majority of Turkish girls nowadays sneak out. But my mum has been brought up more modern, she's sneaked us out to a disco one or two times, without my dad knowing. He'll let us out but my friends have to come round to be looked over and he prefers girls who have got the same background as me. He wouldn't ever let me go to disco because it's late hours, although I can go to the cinema with a girlfriend. He prefers me to go out with my sister, and I prefer it too, I feel more secure. We've only got a year between us. I trust her, we're like best friends, and it doesn't come like that for everyone. You can always break up with a friend but I don't think you can break up with a sister, even though we have fights. I always tell my sister whatever happens and she tells me too.

We were always brought up to know that sex before marriage wasn't acceptable, and so I think if you feel strongly for a boy it's all right, but I don't believe in sex before marriage myself, I'd still prefer to wear my white dress. I don't always agree with my parents but I respect their traditions, so I wouldn't rebel. I'm more into my education. It's not worth doing it just for the experience. Most of my English friends look so depressed and bored. I think it's because they've got so much freedom. They've gone out with boys and slept with them at the age of fifteen and they're not very happy. Everyone's got problems; if it's not sex it's something else. I think I'm lucky. I'm well off, I'm not being beaten or anything.

"Voices from Home", Sue Sharpe, Virago Upstarts 1990

Gillian

All of us children apart from two of my sisters are Catholics. To us religion means everlasting life. It's something that you don't have to practise, it's always there. God is everywhere. If there's something in the Catholic religion that I don't believe in, when I'm at church I back down on these things. For example, no child should be aborted, you mustn't go on the pill, and you can't get married more than once. I don't believe in it really. You're not supposed to hurt another person. That's true, I believe that, but why bring another person into the world if you are going to hurt them? Going on the pill is preventing all the trouble but in our religion it's a disgrace. The older people in church make it sound like it's really wrong.

"Speaking Out", Audrey Osler, Virago Upstarts 1989

Trip to Jam Down
Marcia Chevers

Jamaican parents are also very strict towards their children, not all of them but most of them. When I was there I wore lipstick and a bit more make-up than usual. When one of my aunties noticed she began to tell me off and asked if I thought I was a woman or something. I suppose this was a reflection of her strong religious attitudes. I explained that our way of living in Britain is completely different and told her that if a girl of fifteen and upwards were to wear make-up in England no-one would really say anything, and it is actually quite common for a girl of that age to wear it.

A lot of young girls in Jamaica have babies very early, from the age of thirteen upwards. A few boys asked me if I weren't going to have one and were quite surprised really when I answered, 'no.' One or two of them even went to the extreme of asking me if they could 'breed' me so that they could be the father of my baby. I thought it quite strange that they were not allowed to wear make-up, but when it came to getting pregnant, which is a more serious matter, it was not looked upon so seriously.

"Our lives, Young Peoples Autobiographies", 1979, ILEA English Centre.

Cheryl

My stepdad abused me sexually and physically – by touching me, or he used to beat me when my mum wasn't there. First of all he was only hitting me; then I started hitting him back and he didn't like it. In the end I was provoking him because I was getting sick of him beating me and I was getting cheeky and answering back. I wasn't going to get hit for nothing. When I started screaming he used to cover my mouth, and that's when he sexually abused me. My mum used to go to bingo in the evenings and I remember him making me touch him. I was only six. And when Mum was expecting Lucy it got worse, and then we moved and I just felt relief. When she got pregnant again I hated her because it happened again. She wondered why I was always rebelling against her and him, but I could never say anything although I wanted to tell her.

"Voices from Home", Sue Sharpe, Virago Upstarts 1990

SECTION 3: SEX EDUCATION

ACTIVITY SHEET 25

Different values

MY EXPERIENCE IN THE EASTERN WORLD

In Pakistan a man is thought of being at a higher standard than a woman. From the minute you are born, the treatment you get differs. If you are a boy you will be congratulated and everybody will be happy for you but if a girl is born in the family, then you will get sympathy and condolences. Boys are allowed a lot more freedom than girls. Boys are encouraged to study and take up a good profession, whereas girls are not encouraged to go to school but they are encouraged to learn how to cook and clean and look after your house and husband and become a good wife (not a doctor). While I was in Pakistan I attended a wedding which really surprised me. The girl that was to be married hadn't even seen her future husband. This would rarely take place in England.

It is true that the things I have written about don't take place that often in England but in my community many of these things do happen. Socialising with boys could start rumours and parents are reluctant to let their daughter go out with anyone. Maybe it isn't as bad as it is in Pakistan but it does happen in our community. Our customs, religious beliefs and traditions prevent us from choosing our own husband, socialising with boys etc, but it isn't as bad. For example, my mum got a good friend of mine married (her parents were abroad). It is true that we chose the boy but we didn't just get her married, we let her talk to the boy, go out with him and only after her consent did we get her married. In Pakistan she would be lucky to get a photograph of him!

Salima Nanji
GEN Magazine, issue 9, 1986

Colour Prejudice

Black boy meets white girl, they hold hands,
At this touch Cupid's arrow lands,
But arrow in the front, or in the back,
It doesn't matter, he's still black.
Her parent's give the black a miss, –
That, my friend, is Prejudice.

White boy meets black girl, holds her hand,
Visions of a promised land,
Takes her home to see his dad,
Surprise, surprise, his father's glad,
Her mum likes him as well, you know.
Very strange, even so.
This way round they're not dismissed –
Again, my friend, that's Prejudice.

Peter Williams
"City lines", poems by London School Students, ILEA English Centre, 1982

LAI

Lai is fifteen and lives in the London suburbs with her parents, who came here from Hong Kong with her two elder brothers.

I haven't had a boyfriend but I really want one, although I'm a bit scared. If my mum and dad found out I'd been clubbing they'd think a boy was involved, so they would probably stop me from ever going out again. They think if I have a boyfriend I'll jump into bed with him. But I won't, I just want someone to talk to. I said to Mum, do you think that I can have a boyfriend, and she said when you're seventeen or eighteen – another three years! I really envy English girls sometimes, they can go out without having an excuse, they can have boyfriends, and here's me, always having to wait. I think that's how my mum was brought up. She didn't tell me about the facts of life. When I first started my periods I was eleven and I didn't know what it was. I thought I'd got a serious disease.

My mum is quite religious, we don't have to do everything but she goes to Chinese festivals and worships the gods and whatever. They're Buddhists. I don't really understand it. They don't force me to their religion, but they feel that if you do anything wrong God will be watching you and will punish you and send you to hell. Mum says, "If you sleep with a man before marriage, God won't like it. If you do anything wrong, you'll go to hell." It really scares me. She wants me to have sex after marriage, so she tries to scare me that way. But I think if someone comes at the right time I will, not because I have to lose my virginity but because I love this person. I just won't tell them. But I'm not going to wait until after I'm married. My brothers have done it, so why can't a girl? I point out to her about my decisions and I go, "Do you mind if I marry whatever nationality?" and she says, "Whatever makes you happy," but I think she would prefer me to marry a Chinese man.

"Voices from Home",
Sue Sharpe, Virago Upstarts 1990

SECTION 3: SEX EDUCATION

ACTIVITY 26 Assumptions

Purpose • To explore stereotypes of men and women

Time needed 30 minutes

What you need A copy of Activity Sheet 26, cut in half, for each student. Extra copies of the complete activity sheet for each group of six. Pens. A large piece of flipchart paper or board on which you should write the adjectives which are on Activity Sheet 26.

How you do it
1. Give each student a copy of the top half of Activity Sheet 26. Ask them to fill it in as quickly as they can. Once finished, they should turn it face down.
2. Repeat the process with the bottom half of Activity Sheet 26.
3. Form the students into groups of six. Give each group an unused complete activity sheet and ask them to collate on it the answers from everyone in their group by putting B next to any adjective ticked by a boy, and G next to any ticked by a girl.
4. Collect in all the responses from groups. From them, build a composite list on the flipchart paper or board.

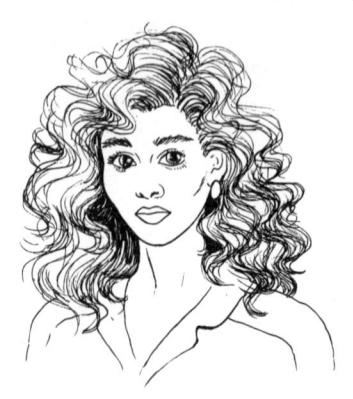

Select one adjective from each pair below which you think applies to the picture of the woman.

G	Confident	Frightened
B	Soft	Hard
G	Intelligent	Stupid B
G	Warm	Cold B
G	Clean	Dirty
B	Dull	Exciting
	Worried	Unworried G B
	Strong	Weak B G
	Dangerous	Safe
G B	Friendly	Unfriendly

Processing questions
- Are there any obvious differences in the adjectives which they thought applied to the man and to the woman?
- Are there any differences in the answers of boys and girls in the group?
- What are some of the assumptions being made?

Suggestions for follow-up work Make a collage of how wo/men are portrayed in the media. Activity 7 explores stereotypes of men and women in advertisements.

SECTION 3: SEX EDUCATION

Assumptions

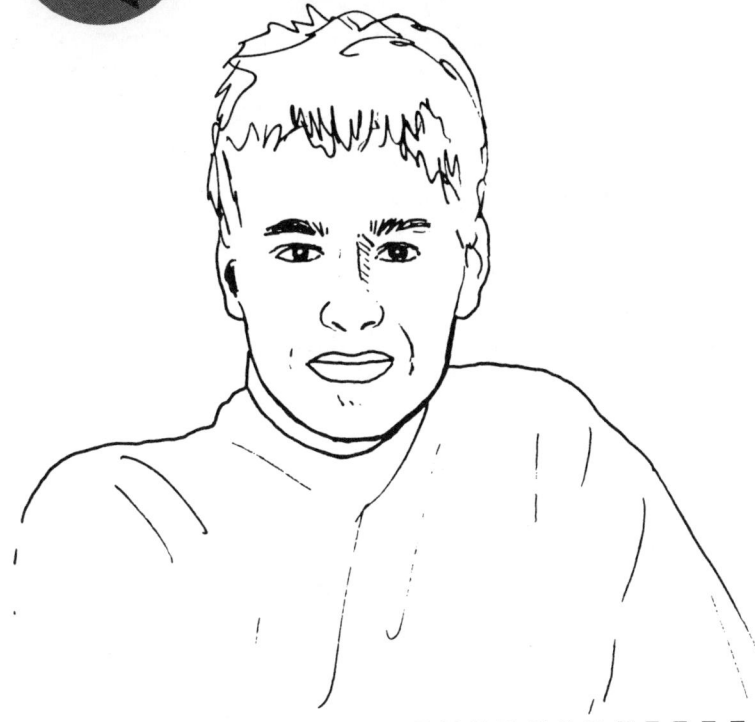

ACTIVITY SHEET 26

Select one adjective from each pair below which you think applies to the picture of the man.

Confident	Frightened
Soft	Hard
Intelligent	Stupid
Warm	Cold
Clean	Dirty
Dull	Exciting
Worried	Unworried
Strong	Weak
Dangerous	Safe
Friendly	Unfriendly

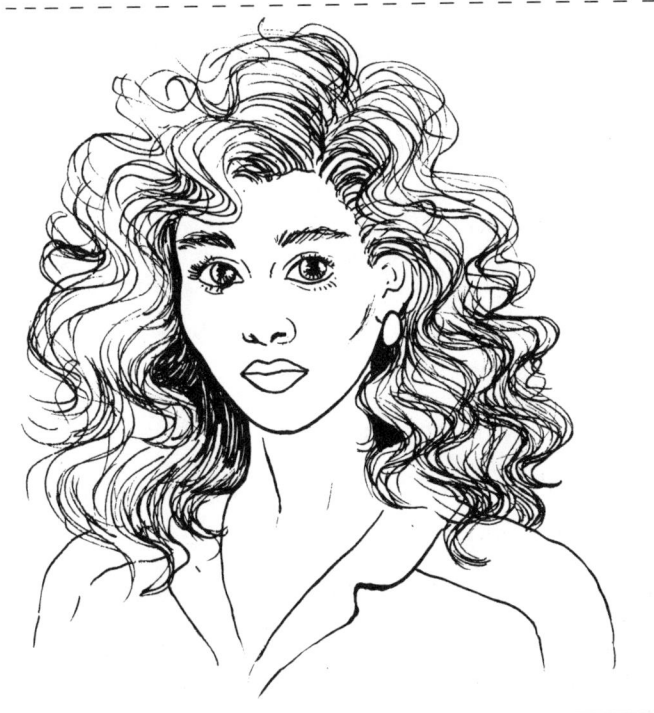

Select one adjective from each pair below which you think applies to the picture of the woman.

Confident	Frightened
Soft	Hard
Intelligent	Stupid
Warm	Cold
Clean	Dirty
Dull	Exciting
Worried	Unworried
Strong	Weak
Dangerous	Safe
Friendly	Unfriendly

© A Picture of Health   Permission to photocopy this page for participant use

Section 3: Sex Education

Activity 27 — Love songs

Purpose
- To use popular songs to encourage discussion
- To explore views on love and sex

Time needed 20 minutes

What you need A short tape of either current chart successes which feature love, romance and sex (which means most!) or some well-known 'golden oldies'. Flipchart or board.

How you do it
1. Divide the group in half.
2. Play the tape, asking one half to listen for any mention of love, the other to listen for any mention of sex. Ask them to think about what sort of attitudes are being expressed in the songs.
3. Write the word 'LOVE' on the flipchart paper or on the board. Ask the half of the group who were focusing on the word 'love' to call out any words or expressions associated with love in the pop songs. Then widen it to any words or expressions which come into their heads when they generally hear the word.
4. Repeat with the other half of the group and the word 'SEX'.
5. Ask the class to look for similarities and differences in the two lists.

Processing questions
- Are pop songs about the real world?
- Are the words in the songs important? Do they influence how we behave?
- How do their own attitudes compare with the ones in the songs?
- What's the difference between 'falling in love' and 'loving'?
- Is there any point in sex without love or love without sex?
- How can you show you love someone without having sex with them?

Suggestions for follow-up work Working in small groups, give each group a different card with one of the following options written on it: going around in a group with no special partner, kissing and holding hands with a girl/boyfriend, heavy petting but not going 'all the way', having unsafe sex (without a condom), having sex with a condom. Ask them to list the advantages and disadvantages of each option.

SECTION 3: SEX EDUCATION

ACTIVITY 28 — *Problem pages*

Purpose
- To discuss relationship problems
- To identify possible strategies to resolve them

Time needed 30–40 minutes

What you need A selection of letters from problem pages of magazines or comics aimed at the students' age group. Choose problems about relationships. Separate each letter from the reply, numbering each so that you can easily match them later. Pens. Paper.

How you do it
1. Give each student a letter.
2. Divide the class into groups of three. Ask each person to read out their letter to the other two. The group is then to choose one letter from their three that particularly interests them.
3. Ask each group to make a list of *everything* they think the writer could do, then decide on and underline the three best options. Get them to discuss how easy or difficult it would be to carry out these three solutions. How would the letter writer need to feel? What would s/he need to be able to do? What might the results be?
4. Ask each group the number of their problem and give them the corresponding answer. Now ask them to compare how the answer compares with their own responses.

Processing questions
- How easy or difficult do they think it would be for the letter writer to solve her/his problem?
- What were some of the best solutions which they identified?
- Were the replies from the magazines similar to their own?
- Why do people write to magazines with their problems? Who else could they turn to? What are the advantages and disadvantages of each source of help?

Suggestions for follow-up work Organise a group project to compile a list of agencies and organisations, including telephone help lines, which offer help to young people. These could be both local and national.

Section 3: Sex Education

Activity 29 — Who'd fall for that line?

Purpose	• To identify the common 'lines' used to pressurise young women, and to a lesser extent men, into sexual activity • To consider assertive responses to these lines
Time needed	30 minutes
What you need	Large sheets of paper. Felt-tip pens. Copies of Activity Sheet 9 or similar materials which define assertiveness.
How you do it	1. Divide the class into small single-sex groups of three or four and give each group a large sheet of paper. 2. Ask each group to write down all the lines they have ever heard which boys use to pressurise girls into sexual activity. Examples might be 'Everyone else is doing it', 'If you love me, you'll do it' and 'Now you've got me going, it's not fair to stop.' 3. After a few minutes, students feed back their lines. Draw up a master list. 4. Ask the students, working in the same groups, to choose one or two lines which they think would be difficult to handle and to think of as many responses as possible. Ask them to record these on the sheet of paper. 5. Hand out Activity Sheet 9 on assertiveness. Ask them to consider which of their responses are assertive. 6. In the whole group, get them to share what they consider to be the most appropriate response.
Processing questions	• Which lines did they think it would be most difficult to handle? • Why do boys use these lines? • Are there any ways in which boys are pressurised into having sex when perhaps they do not want to? (eg, one boy to another, 'Haven't you done it yet?') • What might be the outcome of the responses they identified? • How does it feel to be rejected? • How is the girl likely to feel afterwards if she gives in? • What are the main things to bear in mind in deciding whether to become sexually active in a relationship?
Suggestions for follow-up work	A carousel role play, as in Activity 54, would give students an opportunity to practise responding.

Section 3: Sex Education

Activity 30 — *What's in a word?*

Purpose
- To explore the different words used in talking about sex, particularly parts of the body and sexual intercourse
- To show that different groups feel comfortable with different words
- To identify a language that students will feel comfortable working with
- To illustrate attitudes revealed in language

Time needed 30 minutes

What you need Flipchart paper and pens. Ideas for words – suggestions: vagina, penis, sexual intercourse, contraception, pregnancy.

How you do it
1. Explain to students that if they are going to talk about sexuality, they need to understand medical terms and words commonly used. Point out that it is normal and acceptable to feel uncomfortable with certain sexual words and expressions.
2. Divide the class into groups of three or four. Give each group a sheet of flipchart paper and ask them to find a comfortable working space.
3. Give each group a word (the same as or different from those given to other groups) and ask them to brainstorm all the other words they know with a similar meaning.
4. Re-form as a large group and get them to share the results.

Processing questions
- Which words might be used with/by different people – for example a doctor, a young child, young people with each other, women, men?
- Are there any words which they don't like or which make them feel upset or angry?
- Are there any differences in the way girls/boys react to certain words?
- What sort of attitudes to wo/men are revealed in the words or expressions?
- How did they feel doing this activity?

Suggestions for follow-up work Ask students to find out the definitions of the following words and terms, used in talking about HIV/AIDS:

antibody	homosexual
bisexual	immune system
deficiency	intravenous
HIV	transmission.
heterosexual	

SECTION 3: SEX EDUCATION

Activity 31
Is it true?

Purpose
- To check students' level of knowledge of sexual issues
- To provide accurate information about sexual issues

Time needed   30 minutes

What you need   A copy of Activity Sheet 31A or 31B for each student (31A is general, 31B concentrates on HIV/AIDS). Pens.

How you do it
1. Give each student a copy of the activity sheet chosen. Ask them to work in pairs.
2. Explain that the quiz is for their own use, not a test to be passed or failed.
3. Ask them, working in pairs, to answer the questions in the spaces provided.
4. When everyone has finished, read out the correct answers and ask them to correct their own papers.
5. Encourage a discussion in the whole group.

Processing questions
- Which questions were they both most unsure about?
- Did any of the answers surprise them?
- Would they like more information about any of the answers?
- Where could they get the information?

Suggestions for follow-up work
- Give each student a piece of paper. Ask them to write down a question which they would like answered. They should not put their names on the papers. Collect these in. You can then use these for planning further sessions. For example, you could go through them, taking out any duplicates and combining where possible. If you are left with several on one particular theme, write them out on separate index cards. Proceed as in Activity 32.
- Organise a group project to compile a list of agencies and organisations where young people could get further information. These could be local and national. Students research the type of information and help which each of these can give.

SECTION 3: SEX EDUCATION

ACTIVITY SHEET 31A

Is it true?

Are these statements true or false?

	TRUE	FALSE
1 'Puberty' comes from a word meaning 'to become hairy'		
2 If a girl hasn't started her periods by the age of 14, there's something wrong		
3 At puberty new glands become active and you sweat more		
4 Masturbating or playing with yourself does no harm		
5 All women have a period every twenty-eight days		
6 You can use a tampon if you're a virgin		
7 PMT is a type of contraceptive		
8 There's nothing you can do about painful periods		
9 You have to wait until you've missed two periods to find out if you're pregnant		
10 Making love doesn't always mean sexual intercourse		
11 You can't get pregnant the first time you have intercourse		
12 A woman can't get pregnant if the man withdraws his penis before ejaculating (coming)		
13 The condom is the only method of contraception which gives some protection against HIV, the virus which causes AIDS		
14 You can't tell if someone is infected with the HIV virus just by looking at them		
15 If you have a discharge then you have an STI (a sexually transmitted infection)		
16 It is quite normal for sperm to come out of the penis at night, during sleep		

© A Picture of Health   Permission to photocopy this page for participant use

SECTION 3: SEX EDUCATION

ACTIVITY SHEET 31A

Answer sheet

1 FALSE   'Puberty' comes from the Latin word 'puber', meaning adult. Girls on average reach puberty two years earlier than boys, but everyone develops at their own rate and over several years. Growing hair under your arms and pubic hair is just one change that occurs. By the way, boys may or may not develop hair on their chest, shoulders or lower back. It does not make them any more or less of a man.

2 FALSE   When a girl reaches puberty, she will start to menstruate (or have periods). It is perfectly normal for this to happen any time between the ages of 9 and 15.

3 TRUE   The sweat rate increases and glands in the armpits become active. Also the glands in your skin begin to produce more oil than your skin needs. This affects boys more than girls as it is male hormones which cause the problem. Careful washing of yourself and your clothes is important.

4 TRUE   It can be very pleasurable and is a way of helping you to get to know your own body. Many men and women, with or without partners, enjoy masturbating throughout their lives and consider it as normal, healthy sexual behaviour. Some disagree, thinking it is wrong. They feel that sexual behaviour should be an expression of love between two people and not a one-person act.

5 FALSE   The monthly cycle varies in different women and may be as short as eighteen days or longer than twenty-eight. Most young women just starting to have periods will not have a regular cycle. A cycle begins on the first day of bleeding and ends the day before the start of the next menstrual flow. A period generally lasts from three to seven days.

6 TRUE   A wide range of tampons and sanitary towels are now available, including slim-line tampons designed for young girls. They should be changed regularly, at least every four hours, as they are an ideal culture medium for bacteria.

7 FALSE   PMT stands for 'pre-menstrual tension'. This is a term for the symptoms women may get before a period (eg feeling depressed or moody, headaches, tiredness, tender breasts, feeling bloated). It has been suggested that a lack of the hormone progesterone in the second part of the menstrual cycle may be one of the causes.

© A Picture of Health   Permission to photocopy this page for participant use

Section 3: Sex Education

8 FALSE Exercise, a hot-water bottle or a warm bath can help, as can pain-killers that you buy over the counter. If the pain persists, you should consult your doctor.

9 FALSE Most tests are done when the period is two weeks late. An early-morning sample of urine is tested to see if there is a hormone in it which is present during pregnancy. You can get a test at a family planning clinic, Brook Advisory Centre, pregnancy advice centre and at some chemists. If you go to a doctor, it may take a few days for the results to arrive as the urine sample will be sent to a hospital for testing. You can also buy home pregnancy testing kits from a chemist, although they are quite expensive and are not always reliable if you don't use them correctly.

10 TRUE There are many ways, apart from sexual intercourse, to express affection for someone. Cuddling, kissing and touching can be a very sexy experience and can help people express how they feel about one another. Talking and sharing feelings are other ways to let someone know you care.

11 FALSE There are 200,000 unplanned pregnancies occurring every year to people who say they thought it would not happen the first time. Whenever you have sexual intercourse, especially without contraception, you run the risk of becoming pregnant.

12 FALSE The penis gives off a fluid containing sperm before ejaculation. Sperm in this fluid can result in pregnancy.

13 TRUE It greatly lessens the chance of infection from HIV or any other sexually transmitted diseases.

14 TRUE HIV, the human immuno-deficiency virus, is carried in the blood stream of an infected person. Most people will look perfectly healthy.

15 FALSE Not necessarily. It is normal for a woman's vagina to have a slight discharge at different times in the monthly cycle. Only if it itches or smells bad might there be an infection.

16 TRUE Sperm can be ejaculated spontaneously during sleep, especially during puberty. This release of sperm is called a 'wet dream' or a nocturnal emission.

Section 3: Sex Education

ACTIVITY SHEET 31B — *Is it true?*

How much do you know about HIV/AIDS?
Are these statements true or false?

	TRUE	FALSE
1 AIDS stands for acquired immune deficiency syndrome		
2 If you only have sex with people you know, you won't become infected by HIV		
3 Taking drugs will give you HIV		
4 Babies can be born with HIV		
5 You cannot get HIV from kissing		
6 HIV is difficult to get except in specific ways		
7 If you stick with one partner, you won't become infected with HIV		

SECTION 3: SEX EDUCATION

ACTIVITY SHEET 31B

Answer sheet

1. **TRUE** *Acquired* means you get it from someone else. *Immune deficiency* means your body cannot defend itself against certain illnesses. *Syndrome* means a collection of signs and symptoms which a doctor may recognise as a disease

2. **FALSE** Knowing someone well doesn't mean they don't have an HIV infection

3. **FALSE** Taking drugs will give you HIV only if you inject, using a needle contaminated with HIV

4. **TRUE** Mothers who have HIV can pass it on to their unborn babies

5. **TRUE** There is no evidence of transmission through saliva

6. **TRUE** HIV, which causes AIDS, is only passed on in very specific ways:
   a) close sexual contact (intercourse and, to a lesser extent, oral sex)
   b) by infected blood getting into another person's body
   c) from an infected mother to her unborn or newly born child.

   You cannot get HIV by kissing, hugging, shaking hands, sharing a cup, sitting next to somebody, using the same toilet or swimming in pools.

7. **FALSE** This depends on what your partner did before you met, and on whether either of you has unprotected sex with someone else or injects drugs using dirty needles

Section 3: Sex Education

Activity 32: Contraception

Purpose
- To identify information which students would like about contraceptive methods
- To encourage them to find the information and present it to others

Time needed Depends on the size of the group and the number of questions generated – at least 30 minutes. It could be divided into two sessions.

What you need Leaflets and articles giving information about contraceptive methods. Activity Sheet 32 gives some facts. Further information is available from your local health promotion unit, the Family Planning Association, doctors' surgeries, family planning clinics, magazines and libraries. The same method is applicable to a range of health issues, for example sexually transmitted infections and healthy eating, as long as you have access to printed materials about the issue. Pencils. Index cards.

How you do it

1. Point out that there are several ways of avoiding becoming pregnant. Ask them to call out any which they have heard of and write these on the board. Dispel any which are myths, such as 'Doing it standing up' or 'Using clingfilm', without causing embarrassment to the person who suggested it.
2. Give each student a pencil and an index card.
3. Explain that this session is about contraceptive methods, but that you don't want to go over things which they already know. Ask each person to think of some factual information which they would like about contraception. Keeping it as specific as possible, they should write it in question form, in capital letters, on their index card. An example such as 'How does the morning-after pill work?' might be useful.
4. Collect in the cards, shuffle them and ask each person in turn to take one from the top. If they find it is their own card, tell them to put it back at the bottom of the pile.
5. Give each student a copy of Activity Sheet 32. Working in pairs, each pair should try to find the answer to their two questions in the information on the activity sheet or in other sources which you have made available.
6. After 15 minutes, get them to reform as a group. Ask one pair to read out one of their questions and any information which they have found to answer it. Any pair with a similar question should take a turn next and compare their reply.

SECTION 3: SEX EDUCATION

Processing questions
- How difficult was it to think of a question?
- Was anyone tempted to write something funny? Why might this be?
- Was it easy to find the information needed?
- What did they think of the way in which the information is written? Was it easy to understand?
- Where can people go for more information?

Suggestions for follow-up work
- Get students to devise leaflets which contain the type of information wanted by their age group, in a language and style that they think appropriate.
- Ask them to carry out a research project to find any missing information.

Section 3: Sex Education

Contraception

ACTIVITY SHEET 32

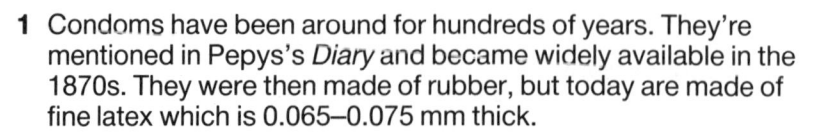

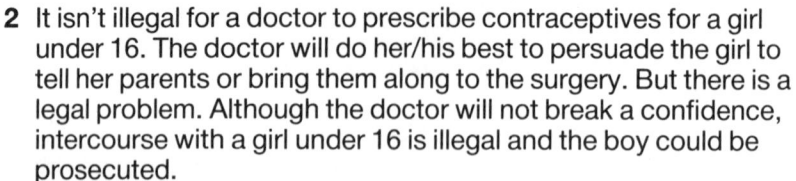

More than fifteen things you might need to know about
CONTRACEPTION

1. Condoms have been around for hundreds of years. They're mentioned in Pepys's *Diary* and became widely available in the 1870s. They were then made of rubber, but today are made of fine latex which is 0.065–0.075 mm thick.

2. It isn't illegal for a doctor to prescribe contraceptives for a girl under 16. The doctor will do her/his best to persuade the girl to tell her parents or bring them along to the surgery. But there is a legal problem. Although the doctor will not break a confidence, intercourse with a girl under 16 is illegal and the boy could be prosecuted.

3. Some people make a deliberate choice not to be involved in sexual relationships with others, either for a short time in their lives or permanently. They may not feel ready for a long-term commitment. This may be a real test of a person's maturity: it can be difficult to resist pressure from people your own age, from the media or from someone you care about. Not having sexual intercourse is the only sure way to avoid pregnancy and sexually transmitted infections.

4. Methods of contraception work in two different ways. There are those which stop the man's sperm from coming into contact with the woman's egg (barrier methods) and those which prevent the egg from settling in the womb (eg the pill).

5. The pill is 99% effective against pregnancy, if taken properly. This means taking it every day, never missing once. It gives no protection whatsoever against sexually transmitted infections such as HIV, the virus which causes AIDS.

6. You shouldn't use the same condom twice.

7. There are many names for condoms: sheath, french letter, Johnny, rubber, the brand names Mates and Durex . . . but don't ask for them by the last name in Australia or you'll be given sellotape!

8. The rhythm method or 'safe period' is based on the fact that during a certain part of the menstrual cycle a woman is less likely to get pregnant. However it is quite difficult to work out, especially for young girls with irregular periods, and is therefore not very safe. It also offers no protection against sexually transmitted infections. It is the only method allowed by the Roman Catholic Church.

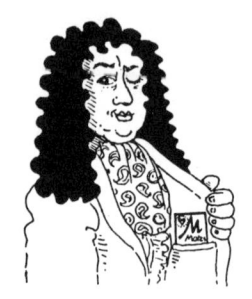

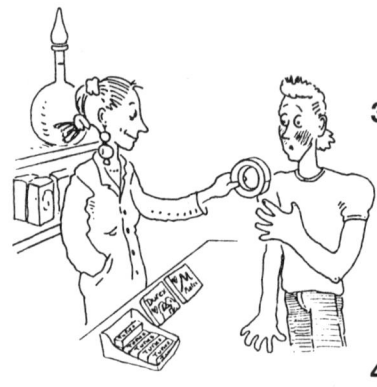

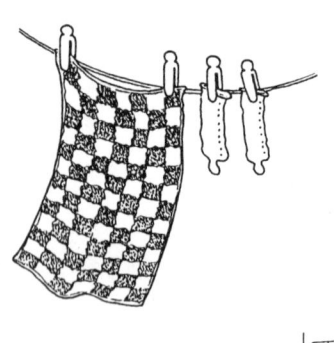

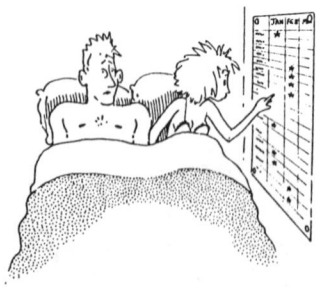

© A Picture of Health   Permission to photocopy this page for participant use

Section 3: Sex Education

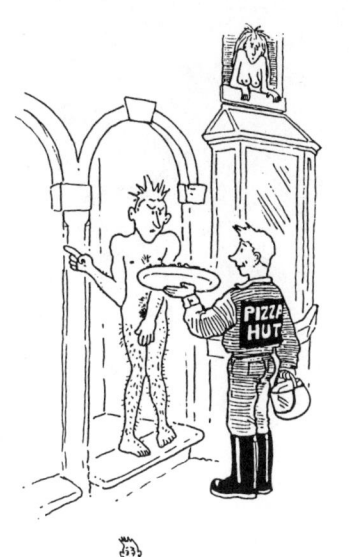

9. Coitus interruptus was once probably the most common form of birth control method, especially by young people first starting intercourse. Other names for it are withdrawal, discharging, pulling out, getting off at Crewe if you are on the way to Glasgow, and being careful. However, it's far from careful! It relies on the man exercising a lot of self-control. A woman may find it hard to relax as she may worry about whether her partner will be as good as his word. A few drops of fluid come out of the penis before a man ejaculates (comes). He has no control over this and that amount of fluid contains millions of sperm. The method offers no protection against HIV.

10. The cap or diaphragm is made of soft rubber and was first devised by a Dutchman called Mensinga in 1885 – which accounts for its other name, Dutch cap. It is put into the vagina before intercourse to cover the cervix (entrance to the womb) and make a barrier which prevents the sperm meeting the egg. It must be used with a spermicidal cream and left in place for 6 hours after intercourse. It has to be fitted initially by a doctor and checked every six months. It may protect a woman against cancer of the cervix, but offers no protection against HIV.

11. Sperm take only 90 seconds to get into the uterus or womb. Methods which rely on getting rid of the sperm quickly – jumping up and down, having sex standing up, coughing, peeing, drinking cold water, douching – are all useless.

12. Certain methods of birth control are permanent and are only suitable for people who are absolutely sure they have completed their family or do not want one at all. These are female sterilisation, when the fallopian tubes are closed so that the egg cannot travel down them to meet the sperm; and male sterilisation or vasectomy, when the tubes through which the sperm travel from the testes to the penis are cut or blocked.

13. Another barrier method is the sponge, which can be bought from chemists. it is a soft, circular, foam sponge containing spermicide. It is put into the vagina up to 24 hours before intercourse and must be left in place for 6 hours afterwards. After removal it's thrown away. Some women may be allergic to the spermicide and it offers no protection against HIV.

14. The IUD stands for intra-uterine device and is commonly known as the coil. It is inserted into the womb by a doctor and is not ideal for a woman who has never been pregnant.

15. It's dangerous to use clingfilm and a rubber band instead of a condom.

16. If you have had sex without using birth control there is an <u>emergency</u> method you can use, the morning-after pill. Treatment must start within three days (72 hours) after sex, the sooner the better. It must be prescribed by a doctor and consists of two special doses of a pill, taken 12 hours apart.

SECTION 3: SEX EDUCATION

ACTIVITY 33 — *Using a condom*

Purpose • To increase awareness about the correct use of condoms

Time needed 30 minutes

What you need Samples of condoms. If time and money permit, make a condom sample book. Buy ten or twelve different types of condom from chemists and supermarkets. Display each as in the illustration, fixing the condom, wrapper and packet with superglue to a sheet of paper and putting these in a display book with transparent plastic wallets (available from stationers). Sets of cards from Activity Sheet 33.

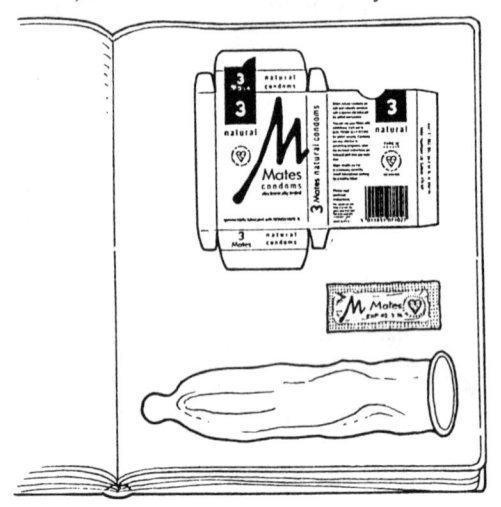

How you do it

1. Point out that the word 'condom' has almost become a household name, but that this doesn't mean that everyone has seen one or knows how to use one properly.
2. Pass round samples of condoms and/or a condom book. Some students may be embarrassed and humour can help to defuse the situation. Some may use the condoms as finger puppets or blow them up like balloons. As long as things don't get out of hand, that can help to release tension. Don't force students to handle condoms against their wishes.
3. Explain that often people do not know how to use a condom effectively. Working in single-sex groups, give each group a set of cards from Activity Sheet 33. Ask them to rearrange these in the correct order.
4. Once they have finished read out the correct answers.

SECTION 3: SEX EDUCATION

Processing questions
- Which cards were the most difficult to place?
- Are there any others which they think should have been included?
- One card which is missing is the woman having an orgasm (or coming). Where do they think that might occur in the order of things? Point out that a woman does not necessarily need penetrative sex to have an orgasm.
- What are the advantages and disadvantages of using a condom?
- Recent surveys have shown that a large number of young people are not taking any notice of the 'safer sex' campaigns to combat AIDS. They are still not using a condom. Why do students think this is? What else can be done to encourage safer sex?

Answers for Activity Sheet 33

12, 4, 1, 8, 7, 13, 5, 6, 3, 9, 14, 11, 2, 10

Section 3: Sex Education

Activity Sheet 33: Using a condom

Photocopy on to card and cut up before use

1 THE PENIS BECOMES HARD/ERECT	**2** TIE KNOT IN CONDOM	**3** THE MAN EJACULATES OR 'COMES'
4 BOTH PARTNERS FEEL TURNED ON OR SEXUALLY EXCITED	**5** UNROLL CONDOM ALL THE WAY DOWN THE PENIS	**6** SEXUAL INTERCOURSE
7 SQUEEZE THE AIR OUT OF THE TIP OF THE CONDOM	**8** OPEN THE PACKAGE	**9** HOLD THE BASE OF THE CONDOM FIRMLY IN PLACE
10 PUT THE CONDOM DOWN THE TOILET OR IN THE BIN	**11** POINT THE PENIS DOWN AND SLIP THE CONDOM OFF	**12** CHECK THE EXPIRY DATE
13 PUT ROLLED-UP CONDOM ON TO TIP OF ERECT PENIS	**14** WITHDRAW THE PENIS IMMEDIATELY BEFORE IT GOES LIMP	

© A Picture of Health   Permission to photocopy this page for participant use

SECTION 4

Family life education

Section 4: Family Life Education

Activity 34 Family roles

Purpose
- To help students understand the many forms a family can take
- To examine a variety of family situations and consider the reasons for different roles and patterns of behaviour in families

Time needed 35 minutes

What you need Large sheets of paper. Coloured felt tip pens.

How you do it
1. Invite students to brainstorm their ideas of different types of family. Allow 3 to 5 minutes, and write down all the words and phrases on a large sheet of paper. Encourage everyone to contribute and to share ideas of what a family is. Does it include the following?
   - Old and young as a family
   - Mixed-race families
   - Childless families
   - Single-parent families
   - Extended families to include communal living, institutions, and residential homes
   - Homosexual families
2. In the whole group, explore with students what they think is the purpose of families. Emphasise that the family meets a range of needs and these may differ in different cultures, for example:
   - Food, shelter and clothing
   - Love and support
   - A means of handing down traditions
   - A way of offering a set of values and beliefs as a framework for how to behave

   Record students' views on a large sheet.
3. Ask each student to make up a funny cartoon strip which shows them and members of their family during a typical Saturday.
4. Display the cartoon strips and encourage students to describe to the others what members of the family are doing.

Processing questions
- Are boys and girls both expected to help with chores?
- Are brothers and sisters treated the same?
- What were the similarities and differences in the ways the class spent their Saturday?
- Are roles in the family fixed or do they change?
- Have the jobs of men and women at home and in the workplace been changing?
- Where do our images about typical roles in the family come from?

Section 4: Family Life Education

Suggestions for follow-up work
- Ask students to watch a family TV series/programme and answer the following questions:
  > How did the men and women behave? (eg were they emotional, aggressive, dependent, confident, brave, shy?)
  > What roles did the men and women take?
  > Which behaviours and roles were traditional and which modern and non-sexist?

  Discuss the findings in the next session.
- Explore different perceptions and experiences of family life. Use literature (prose or poems) which describes family life and is appropriate to the ability and background of your students.

SECTION 4: FAMILY LIFE EDUCATION

ACTIVITY 35 — *The trouble with grown-ups*

Purpose
- To describe different kinds of common family problems
- To identify some ways of solving family conflicts
- To recognise changing relationships within the family
- To practise coping skills for use when problems arise

Time needed 40 minutes

What you need Flipchart. A copy of Activity Sheet 35 for each student. Pens.

How you do it
1. Give each student a copy of Activity Sheet 35 to complete.
2. Invite students to share their answers in pairs.
3. Bring the class together to discuss:
   ○ When is someone 'grown-up'?
   ○ What kind of things bothered them most about grown-ups?
   ○ Was it the same for boys and girls?
   ○ How could things be improved?
4. Brainstorm typical situations that cause arguments in families.
5. Record the suggestions on the flipchart and invite students to work in pairs on one situation of their choice. One person takes one side of the conflict and one the other. Each pair should try to find a way of resolving their conflict.
6. Bring the group together to discuss ways in which family arguments might be resolved.

Processing questions
- What helped and what hindered the argument?
- Was it possible for each person to give their point of view?
- Did people use their listening skills?
- Were they able to say how they felt about the situation?
- Are there times when it is better to keep your feelings to yourself?

Suggestions for follow-up work Ask students to keep a personal diary of arguments/conflicts for one week. They should note down the causes and how they responded to them, then look for ways which helped each party to see the other's point of view.

SECTION 4: FAMILY LIFE EDUCATION

ACTIVITY SHEET 35

Parents and children questionnaire

1. Grown-ups do and say a lot of things that bother or embarrass young people when they are growing up. It can help to share and talk about these things. Complete the sentences below and share your answers or discuss those you want to talk about with a partner.

   I feel puzzled when grown-ups ....

   ....

   I feel disappointed when grown-ups ....

   ....

   I feel appreciated when grown-ups ....

   ....

   I feel confused when grown-ups ....

   ....

   I feel sad when grown-ups ....

   ....

   I feel angry when grown-ups ....

   ....

   I feel embarrassed when grown-ups ....

   ....

   I feel cheerful when grown-ups ....

   ....

© A Picture of Health   Permission to photocopy this page for participant use

Section 4: Family Life Education

2 How do you hope that you will behave with children when you are grown up? List the things you think are important.

....

....

....

....

....

....

3 List three things you would try not to do or say to children when you are grown up.

....

....

....

Section 4: Family Life Education

Activity 36: *Changes*

Purpose
- To stimulate thought and discussion about events connected with the lives of students and their families
- To encourage them to think about what helped or hindered in the changes they encountered
- To help them think positively about the future

Time needed 40 minutes

What you need Large sheet of paper for each student. Coloured crayons or felt-tip pens.

How you do it
1. Give each student a sheet of paper and ask them to draw on it a Timeline from 0 to 15 years. Let them work out a suitable scale and mark the years on it.
2. Each student should think about significant events that have happened in her/his own life that were important to her/him (eg starting nursery school/primary school, the arrival of a brother or sister, having an accident, losing a friend). They should mark these events on their Timeline, either with a small sketch or a symbol. Allow plenty of time for students to fill in their Timeline up to the present.
3. Ask students to share their Timelines with another person. Each should share one or two significant events on their Timeline, saying why it was important. The other person should try to understand and empathise with the one who is talking.
4. When everyone has finished talking about their Timeline, invite students to continue by mapping out an imaginary Timeline for themselves for the next fifty years.

Processing questions
- How easy is it to remember events?
- What kind of things helped them to overcome problems or difficulties at the time?
- How have relationships and responsibilities changed as they grew older?
- Does it help to share experiences with another person?
- Was it easy or difficult to speculate about the future?
- Do we look forward to change?

Suggestions for follow-up work Suggest that students ask a parent or relative to draw up a Timeline and share it with them. This could give them an insight into the way in which lives have changed in the past fifty years or so. It might be possible to build a Timeline with photographs that show the events recorded on it. How do students think events will be recorded in the future?

Section 4: Family Life Education

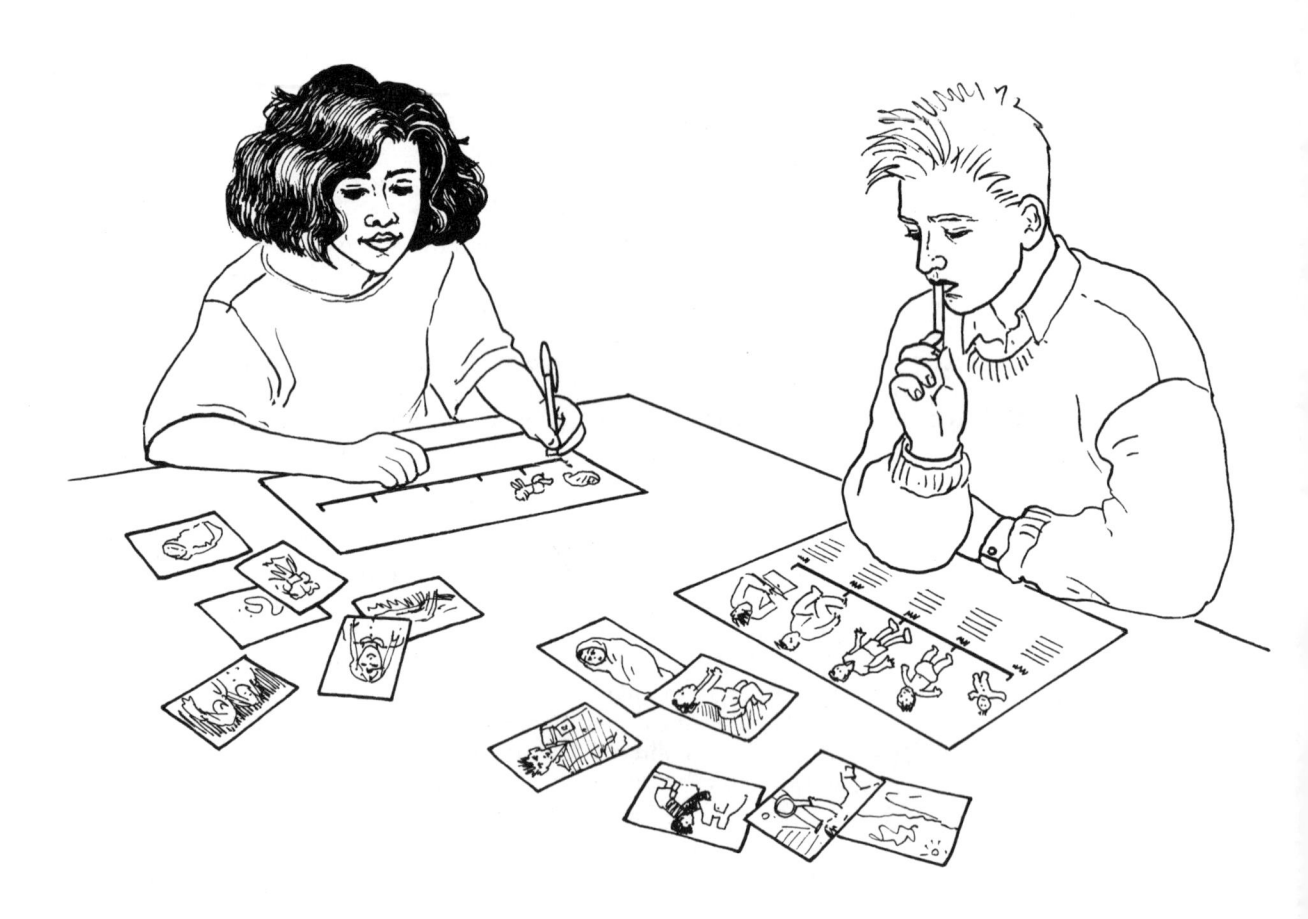

Section 4: Family Life Education

Activity 37 — The needs of children

Purpose
- To identify and share aspects of students' own childhood
- To develop work on the needs of children

Time needed 40 minutes

What you need Sets of photographs of children of different ages – a baby, a toddler, a 6-year-old, a 9-year-old, a young teenager. Paper. Pens.

How you do it
1 Ask students to think about a happy moment from their early childhood and share it with a partner. They should describe to each other what age they were at the time and what made it special.
2 Repeat with students thinking about something that frightened them when they were small. Were their fears imaginary or real? How were they helped to overcome a childhood fear?
3 Bring the class together to talk about their childhood memories. Lead them into a discussion about the needs of children.
4 Ask students to work in groups. Give each group a set of photographs. The group should draw up a list of what they think are the most important needs for the children in the photographs.
5 Display the lists and compare the differences in the needs of the children in the photographs.

Processing questions
- Were there common needs (eg food, warmth, shelter)?
- Are there needs which must be met if children are to develop normally? (eg stimulating play, being talked to, loving care).
- How much do they need other people? Do the people they need change as they grow up?

Suggestions for follow-up work Ask each student to draw up a list of all the good things about being the age they are now. Then get them to make a list of the difficulties. What would make things easier?

SECTION 4: FAMILY LIFE EDUCATION

Activity 38: Coping with loss

Purpose	• To help students understand the feelings associated with loss and separation • To identify ways of dealing with loss
Time	30 minutes
What you need	A copy of Activity Sheet 38 for each student. Pens. Paper.
How you do it	1 Introduce the topic of loss by asking students to look at the people in the pictures on Activity Sheet 38. They have all lost something that is precious to them. Loss touches everyone throughout life: the small child loses a toy; older ones lose friends when they move school; all will experience a big loss when someone close to them dies. The last kind of loss is called **bereavement**. People respond to situations of loss by **grieving**. All changes have an element of loss – when people move on they leave something behind. 2 Ask students to work in pairs and share with each other a time when they lost something or somebody that they loved or needed. Ask them to describe the feelings to their partner. Get them to think about how their feelings changed with time. (It may help to use the circle of feelings chart on Activity Sheet 38.) 3 Invite students to work in groups of five to six to draw up a list of five things that would help a bereaved friend and five things that would not help. How would they choose to help a friend? 4 Bring the class together to discuss the best ways of helping someone to cope with loss. Draw attention to any points from the following list that are not included in the students' lists:
DO	– Be there to listen and stay around – Show you care – Allow the person to express how unhappy they feel – Encourage crying if they want to – Allow them to talk about their loss as often as they like – Help them with everyday things, like schoolwork or shopping
DON'T	– Tell people what they should feel or do – Change the subject when their loss is mentioned – Point out that they have other people or things that matter – Avoid people because of your embarrassment
Suggestions for follow-up work	• Ask students to write a story or poem about sadness. • Point out that one of the qualities needed for helping someone through a loss is the ability to listen. Refer to Activity 23 on listening skills.

SECTION 4: FAMILY LIFE EDUCATION

ACTIVITY SHEET 38 — *Coping with loss*

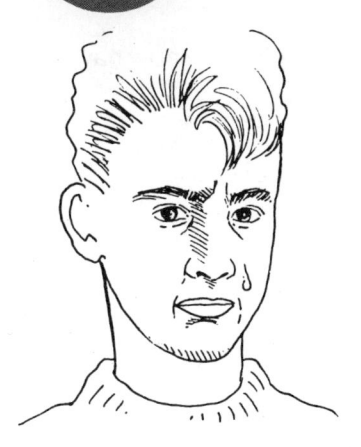

Stan's parents are going to divorce and he may not see one of them very often.

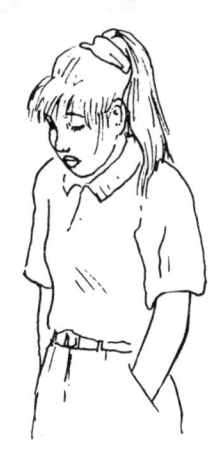

Beth's friend has told her she doesn't want to be her friend any more.

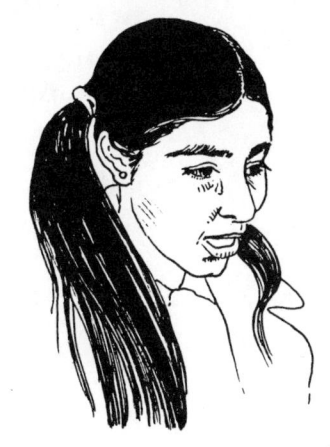

Sulinder's dog was run over and killed.

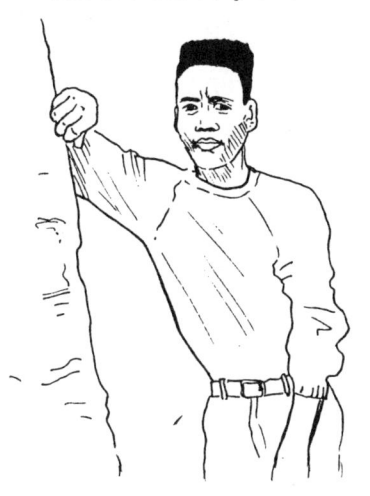

Wesley has to change schools because his parents are moving house.

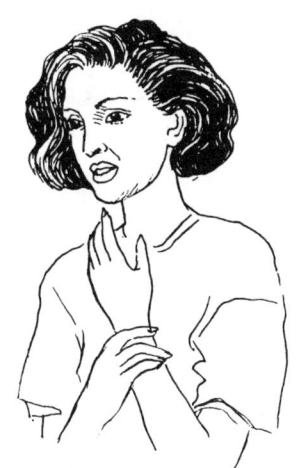

Liz lost her favourite bracelet.

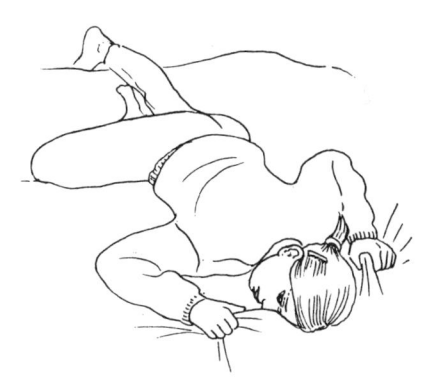

Karen's gran has just died.

Look at the pictures. All of these people have lost something that is precious to them.

Work with a partner. Discuss: . . .
> Have you ever been in a situation like this?
> Can you describe your feelings?

Section 4: Family Life Education

Look at the circle of feelings chart below. This may help you to find the words.

Circle of feelings chart

Circle the feelings you or your partner or people you know have experienced at times of loss.

	Hurt	Helpless	
	Hopeless	Shocked	
Lonely			Guilty
	Disbelieving	Panicky	
Sad			Unhappy
	Vulnerable	Insecure	
Numb			Powerless
	Dazed	Anxious	
Fearful			Tearful
	Tired	Tearful	
	Bewildered	Pained	

SECTION 4: FAMILY LIFE EDUCATION

ACTIVITY 39 — *Looking after children*

Purpose
- To help young people recognise the factors involved in planning and having a family
- To understand what is involved in looking after children

Time 1 hour, plus preparation time for the visit and follow-up afterwards

What you need Parents of young children who have been briefed about the visit. Activity Sheet 39. An outline programme/agenda agreed with the class beforehand. Paper. Pens.

How you do it

Stage 1 – Preparation for the visitors

1 Encourage students to think of young parents they know who might be willing to be the visitors (perhaps young parents among the school community, friends or relations). Once they have been identified, agree on how they will be contacted and on a suitable date and time for the visit.

2 The visitors will need to be fully briefed about the purpose of the visit, the size of the group and the form of the questions.

3 Ask students to work in small groups to decide what kind of questions to ask the visitors. The aim is to find out what is involved in becoming a parent and bringing up children. Bring the whole group together to draw up a final list of questions. If they have difficulty with this, use the following prompts:

  – How did they decide to become parents?
  – What is the most rewarding thing about being a parent?
  – What do they find most difficult?
  – What are the ways in which their lives have changed since becoming parents?
  – How did their friends react to them becoming parents?
  – Do they live near parents/relatives?
  – What, if any, help or support do they have in bringing up their baby/children?
  – How do they share responsibility for looking after their baby/children?
  – What financial pressures are involved in having children?
  – What are the benefits/drawbacks of small or large families?

4 Prepare for the visit, using Activity Sheet 39. Remind students that while personal questions are acceptable in this session, they need to be sensitive to any reluctance to answer and avoid intruding on privacy.

Stage 2 – The visit

1 A member of staff may chair the visit, but students should take responsibility for meeting the visitors, making them feel welcome and ensuring each contributor plays her/his part.
2 Afterwards, review the visit with students.

Processing questions
- How well did they cope?
- Did the visitors seem happy and at ease?
- Was there anything they might have done differently?
- What did they learn about being the parents of young children?
- Is there anything they want to discuss further?
- How realistic are the pictures of family life we get on TV and in the media?

Suggestions for follow-up work
- Ask each student to try to choose a young child that s/he knows well for study; this could be a brother or sister. They should write a description of a typical day in the child's life. Questions they should consider are: Who looks after them? What do they eat? Where do they play? What time do they get up and go to bed?
- Get students to write about the advantages and disadvantages of being an only child.

SECTION 4: FAMILY LIFE EDUCATION

ACTIVITY SHEET 39

Preparing for a visitor

These questions will help the class to prepare for the visit. Everyone can be clear about their own contribution.

? Who will meet the visitors?

? How can the group make the visitors feel welcome/relaxed?

? How will the room be arranged?

? Who will ask the first question?

? Are there key questions we would want asked if time is short?

? Is everyone to be involved?

? How can we encourage the visitors to ask questions?

? Who will bring the session to a close?

? Who will offer thanks?

? Who will see the visitors out?

? Do we want to record the visit in any way?

SECTION 4: FAMILY LIFE EDUCATION

ACTIVITY 40 — *Early learning*

Purpose
- To help students to identify the needs of children of different ages
- To offer practical advice for use when looking after children

Time needed 30 minutes

What you need A set of age cards for each group. A copy of Activity Sheet 40 for each student. Flipchart paper.

How you do it
1. Divide the class into groups. Give each group an age card. Tell them they are to imagine they have been asked to look after a child of the age on their card for an afternoon. They are to draw up a checklist of points they think would be important to ask before being left to baby-sit. Ask how they would plan for the afternoon.
2. Bring the groups together. Ask them to discuss their checklists and draw up plans according to chronological age: baby to 6-year-old.

Processing questions
- Were there things in common (eg how to contact the parents in an emergency; telephone numbers of family doctor/neighbour; if, when and how to feed the child; if the child cries, how to reassure it)?
- Did the plans for the afternoon reflect the stage of development and interests of the child? How did they decide what was appropriate?
- Why is play important for children's development?
- How many groups planned to use TV or books to entertain children?

Suggestions for follow-up work
- Arrange a visit to a local nursery or playgroup in order to observe children, or invite someone who runs a playgroup or nursery to the class. Prepare for the visit as in Activity 39.
- Ask students to collect and examine toy catalogues to see what activities/toys are recommended for the different ages. How accurate do they think the catalogues are?

SECTION 4: FAMILY LIFE EDUCATION

ACTIVITY SHEET 40

Early learning

DID YOU KNOW

... a child cannot develop unless it is with other people?

... skills like walking and talking are learned by children throughout the world at roughly the same age, before their second birthday?

... to learn about life, babies need stimulation: brightly coloured toys, listening to rattles and being talked to?

... language is learned by listening and practising sounds? Language is a basic human need. Speaking to a baby or child teaches her/him about communication. A child learns about the world by asking questions. S/he learns to interpret from different tones of voice.

... play activity helps to develop language, physical skills, social behaviour, intellect and imagination?

CAN YOU SUGGEST IDEAS FOR ACTIVITIES APPROPRIATE FOR CHILDREN AT DIFFERENT AGES?

Baby of 3 months ....

....

....

....

1-year-old ....

....

....

....

Section 4: Family Life Education

Toddler ....
....
....
....

4-year-old ....
....
....
....

6-year-old ....
....
....
....

SECTION 5

Safety

Section 5: Safety

Activity 41 — *Are you a risk-taker?*

Purpose
- To explain the concept of risk-taking
- To identify the types of risk common in the lives of young people
- To identify positive and negative aspects of risk-taking

Time needed   30 minutes

What you need   A copy of Activity Sheet 41 for each student. Flipchart or board. Pens.

How you do it
1. Explain that taking risks is part of everyday life and that there can be no learning without taking risks.
2. Ask each student to complete Activity Sheet 41.
3. Ask them to share their answers with a partner. Are they able to identify risks they both take?
4. Bring the group together to discuss what they mean by 'risk'. Is it possible to agree on a definition? (One definition might be: 'The possibility that something unpleasant may happen as a result of an action.') Record all the suggestions made by the group on a flipchart or board.
5. Brainstorm all the reasons there might be for taking risks, for example to achieve a goal they had set themselves, to prove how tough they are, to push their abilities to the limit, to do something for a laugh. Write down the reasons.
6. Ask students to examine the list of reasons put forward and decide what type of risks might be involved. Are they physical risks? Legal risks? Financial risks? Social risks? Psychological risks?

Processing questions
- Are there particular kinds of risks taken by young people?
- Can they think of a time when taking a risk paid off?

Suggestions for follow-up work   Ask each student to choose two or three of the actions on Activity Sheet 41 and to think of the benefits and advantages of taking that action. Get them to share their answers with the whole group.

Section 5: Safety

Activity Sheet 41

Are you a risk-taker?

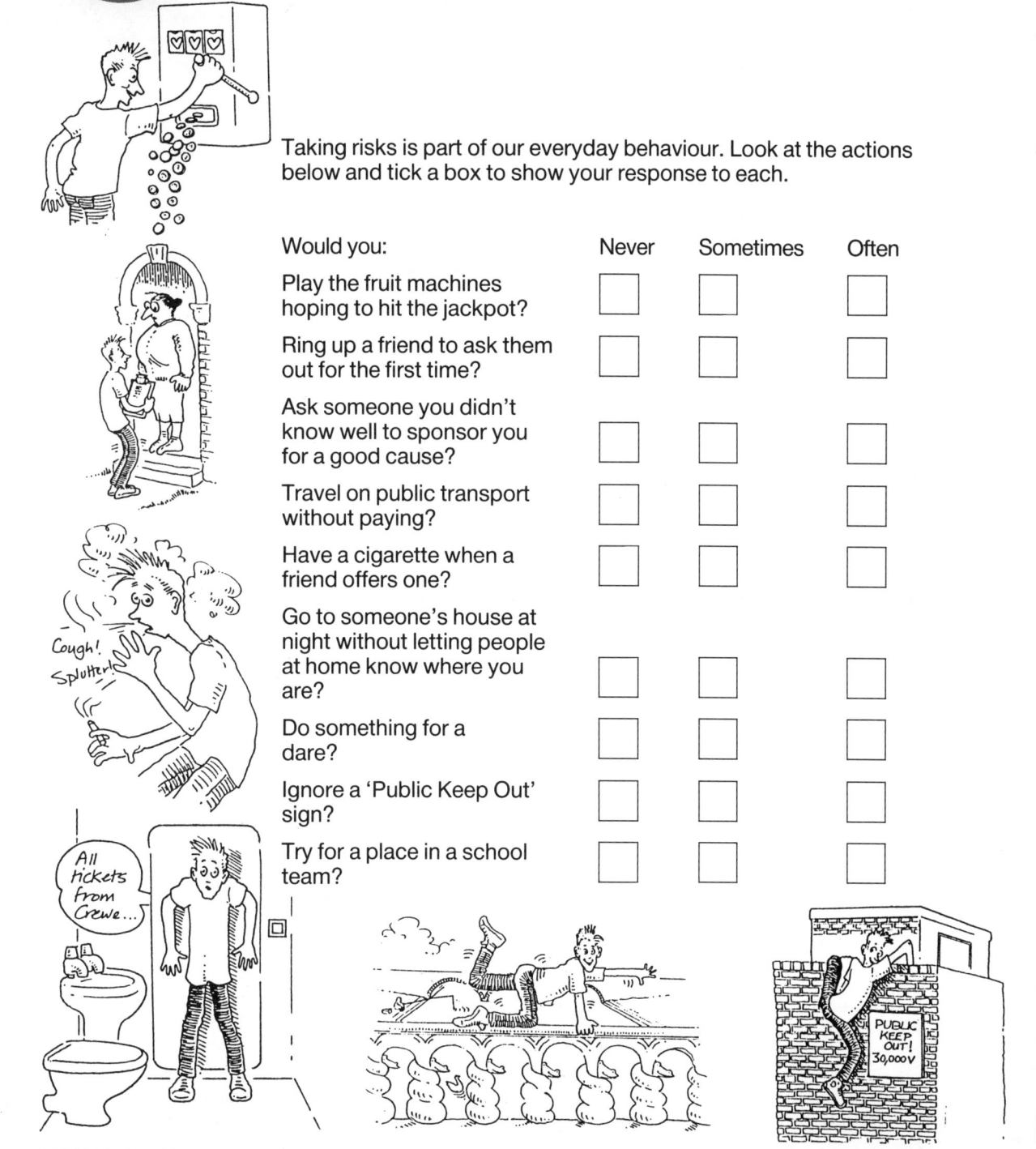

Taking risks is part of our everyday behaviour. Look at the actions below and tick a box to show your response to each.

Would you:	Never	Sometimes	Often
Play the fruit machines hoping to hit the jackpot?	☐	☐	☐
Ring up a friend to ask them out for the first time?	☐	☐	☐
Ask someone you didn't know well to sponsor you for a good cause?	☐	☐	☐
Travel on public transport without paying?	☐	☐	☐
Have a cigarette when a friend offers one?	☐	☐	☐
Go to someone's house at night without letting people at home know where you are?	☐	☐	☐
Do something for a dare?	☐	☐	☐
Ignore a 'Public Keep Out' sign?	☐	☐	☐
Try for a place in a school team?	☐	☐	☐

© A Picture of Health   Permission to photocopy this page for participant use

Section 5: Safety

Activity 42 — *What are the chances?*

Purpose • To show how risk factors can contribute to the chances of developing disease or maintaining health

Time 40 minutes

What you need A set of red chips and a set of white chips (see Activity Sheet 42A). A set of Risk and Healthy Habits cards (see Activity Sheet 42B). The number of each should be equal to half your class plus 10. (Therefore a class of thirty needs twenty-five red and twenty-five white). Two transparent plastic bags. A copy of Activity Sheet 42C for each student. A class of over twenty pupils.

How you do it

1. Explain to students that they are about to play a game in which they will learn more about risk factors, and that a risk factor is a habit or condition associated with an increase in the risk of developing a disease or having an accident.

2. Draw an imaginary line down the middle of the class. Ask one student to hold up a plastic bag in front of each half. In each bag place five red chips, representing illness, and five white chips, representing health.

3. Point out that a person drawing a chip at random from either bag would have a 50:50 chance of drawing a red (illness) or a white (health) chip. Ask students to imagine that these represent the chances of a person developing a disease or staying healthy in the absence of any risk factors. Then point out that in reality people do things that either decrease or increase their chances of staying healthy. Can they think of examples?

4. Place a set of Risk and Healthy habits cards at the front of the class. Ask each student to take a card in turn and read it aloud. If a Risk card is drawn they sit on the left side of the class and put a red chip in the plastic bag. If a Healthy habits card is drawn they sit on the right and put a white chip in the plastic bag.

5. There are now two groups of people: the risk group and the healthy group. Ask for ten volunteers from each group. Each volunteer, in turn, should close her/his eyes and take a chip from the bag belonging to the group. The hope is to draw out a white chip, standing for health. Each group should appoint a score-keeper to add up the total numbers of whites (healthy) and reds (unhealthy) drawn by the group.

6. The group with many risks factors is much more likely to draw red (unhealthy) chips than the other group. The game may need to be

Section 5: Safety

played more than once to demonstrate this as it is possible for students to draw more of the less likely chips in a single round.

7   The total number of red chips will be higher for the group that has accumulated risk factors. It is likely that some students in that group will have drawn white health chips. In the same way on the right-hand side there will be students who drew a red chip. Point out that this is what happens in real life.

8   Give each student a copy of Activity Sheet 42C to read. Bring the group together.

Processing questions
- Can students think of reasons why certain groups of people may be particularly at risk?
- Can they identify ways of reducing risk factors affecting their own health?

Suggestions for follow-up work   Ask students to take Activity Sheet 42C away to discuss with people at home.

Section 5: Safety

ACTIVITY SHEET 42A

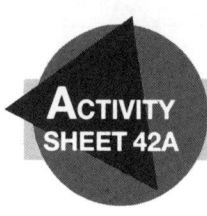

Risk factor game

Photocopy onto card and cut up before use.

To play the game you need twenty more chips than there are students in the class. Take photocopies of this sheet to give you enough chips, colour half red and cut them all out.

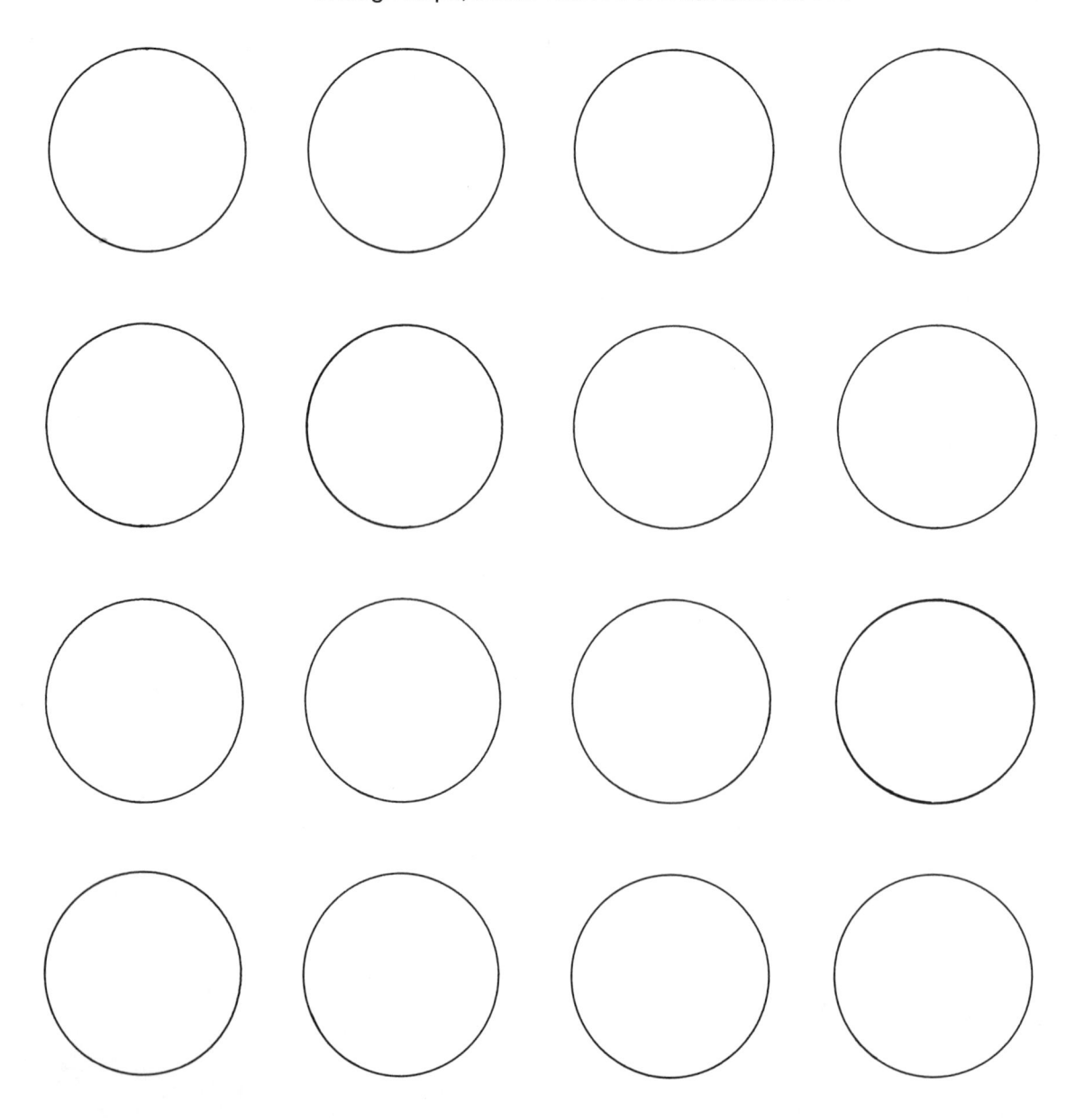

© A Picture of Health   Permission to photocopy this page for participant use

SECTION 5: SAFETY

Cards for a risk factor game

ACTIVITY SHEET 42B

You train after school three times a week. Add a white chip.	You smoke ten cigarettes a day. Add a red chip.	You eat low-fat products and try to cut down on fats in your diet. Add a white chip.
You wear a helmet when you ride a bike. Add a white chip.	You are always very careful when you cross a road. Add a white chip.	You eat lots of fresh fruit. Add a white chip.
You eat lots of greasy foods and creamy puddings. Your risk of gaining weight is high. Add a red chip.	You like to have lots of sugary drinks and sweets. Add a red chip.	You think immunisation is unnecessary. Add a red chip.
You eat breakfast every morning. Add a white chip.	You work with dangerous chemicals. Add a red chip.	There has been a campaign to clean up the environment in your area. Add a white chip.
Your family has a history of heart disease. Add a red chip.	You never drink alcohol and drive. Add a white chip.	You work in an office where a lot of people smoke. Add a red chip.

© A Picture of Health   Permission to photocopy this page for participant use

Section 5: Safety

You work in an office where a lot of people smoke. Add a red chip.	You swim three times a week. Add a white chip.	You take very little exercise. Add a red chip.
You live in an area where the air is heavily polluted. Add a red chip.	After two years of smoking you have given up and haven't had a cigarette for three years. Add a white chip.	You are under a lot of stress and strain and have no one to talk to about it. Add a red chip.
You never eat breakfast in the morning. Add a red chip.	You have friends to talk to when you have a problem. Add a white chip.	You have taken up judo. Add a white chip.
You never get to bed before 11.30pm. Add a red chip.	You are 10lb overweight. Add a red chip.	You stay up late now and again, but generally get enough sleep. Add a white chip.
You always eat wholemeal bread. Add a white chip.	You brush your teeth and gums regularly. Add a white chip.	You never walk to school but go by bus. Add a red chip.

SECTION 5: SAFETY

ACTIVITY SHEET 42C

Stacking the odds

Accumulating a lot of risk factors is like stacking the odds against yourself. Read through the questions and answers below to find out how risk factors can affect your health.

What do risk factors have to do with health?

A risk factor is a habit or condition associated with an increase in our risk of developing a disease or illness. The risk factors for today's major killers – such as coronary heart disease and cancers – include poor dietary habits, lack of exercise, obesity, smoking and environmental pollution. A family history of disease, your age and your gender can also increase or decrease the risk of developing some diseases. Usually more than one risk factor is associated with a disease.

No one in my family has had heart disease or cancer. I'm OK, aren't I?

Heredity is one risk factor you may not have to worry about, but research has shown that smoking, poor dietary habits and lack of exercise are other key risk factors.

My granddad was overweight, ate what he liked, smoked forty cigarettes a day and lived to be 80 years old. Why can't I do the same?

You might get away with it but the odds are stacked against you. Imagine two groups of people, one with lots of risk factors and one with very few. Many more people in the first group will develop health problems than will in the second group. That doesn't mean every single person in the first group gets ill and no one in the second group. It does mean that people who accumulate more risk factors have a greater chance of disability or early death.

My family and I are healthy. I don't see what we need to worry about.

Heart disease, diabetes and many cancers are diseases that build up slowly and invisibly over a long time. Good health habits, established in early life, can stop trouble before it begins.

I don't understand all the fuss. We all die in the end, don't we?

True, but the quality of life is important. Heart attacks, strokes and respiratory diseases don't always kill. Many people are left severely disabled, unable to do what they want when they want, and dependent on others. Good health habits can lead to a fuller, more active life.

Section 5: Safety

Activity 43: Decisions, decisions

Purpose
- To help students recognise the way in which they make decisions
- To offer a decision-making model
- To provide practice in decision-making

Time needed 40 minutes

What you need A copy of Activity Sheets 43A and 43B for each student. Flipchart or board. Pens.

How you do it
1. Give each student a copy of Activity Sheet 43A to complete on their own. Explain that everyone makes decisions in different ways.
2. Ask students to suggest what important decisions face 13- to 14-year-olds. Record their suggestions.
3. Divide the class into groups of four to talk about some important decisions they have to take now or in the future. Ask them to think about who might help them make these decisions. Whose advice might they listen to? What might influence the way they make their choices?
4. Bring the class together to share whom they identified as important in their decision-making processes. Why were those people important? Allow time to discuss the reasons (being listened to, being concerned, being understanding).
5. Explain that it can be helpful to go through a decision-making process when faced with important decisions. Give each student a copy of Activity Sheet 43B. Ask them to decide in groups of three or four on a course of action for each of the situations on the sheet. They can do this by working through the stages suggested to help their decision-making.
6. Bring the class together to review the decisions they made.

Processing questions
- Does it help to recognise what influences us when we make decisions?
- Do we automatically go through the steps of the decision-making process in our heads or does it help to write the steps down?
- Do we rely on making off-the-cuff decisions we may regret later?

Suggestions for follow-up work
- Ask students to identify a decision which they may soon have to make and to apply the steps on Activity Sheet 43B. They could share the results in pairs.
- This activity links with Activities 9 and 10 on assertiveness.

Section 5: Safety

How do you decide?

ACTIVITY SHEET 43A

People make decisions in different ways. We all have favourite approaches. Look at the people in the pictures and see which ones are most like you.

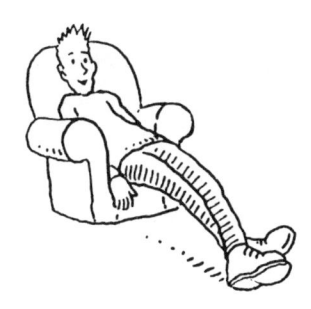

EASY GOING I go along with the rest of the gang.

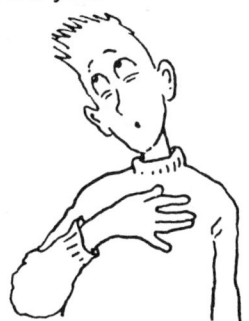

EMOTIONAL Depends on what I feel. I go with my mood.

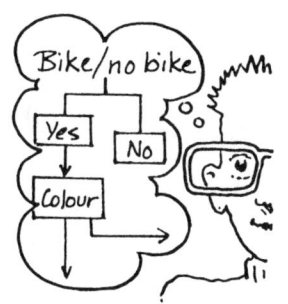

LOGICAL I think things through carefully before I decide.

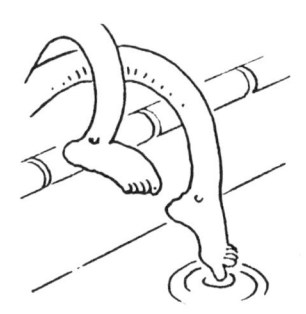

HESITANT I put off deciding as long as I can.

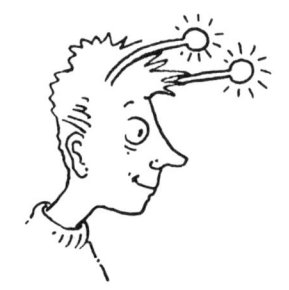

INTUITIVE I know the sort of person I am and I stick to it.

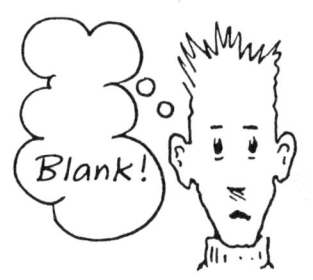

NO THOUGHT I don't like thinking about things too much. I just get on and do it.

There is no one style that is best but certain decisions need particular approaches.

How would you decide on the following:
- Whether to dye your hair?
- Which video to get?
- Whether to go to a disco?
- Whether to buy a new bike?
- Whether to have your ears pierced?
- Whether to have an alcoholic drink at a party?
- Which subjects to choose at school?

Section 5: Safety

List below four or five important decisions you will have to make in your life.

....

....

....

....

....

Section 5: Safety

ACTIVITY SHEET 43B

Making decisions

1
THE SITUATION

8
RECONSIDER

2
THE ALTERNATIVES

7
REVIEW

3
ADVANTAGES/
DISADVANTAGES

6
ACTION

4
THE CHOICE

5
PLAN OF ACTION

When you are making an important decision, following a decision-making process may help. Practise this by applying the suggested steps 1 to 8 to the situations described below.

The steps suggested are:
1. Find out all the facts you want to know about the situation or problem
2. Consider what alternatives are available
3. Think about the advantages/disadvantages of each course of action
4. Choose what to do
5. Make a plan of action
6. Take action
7. Review the choice you made
8. Study the effects of your decision

Choose the situation that interests you most of those outlined below.

Situation A

You have a regular baby-sitting job with the Roberts family on Friday nights. You are saving the money you earn to help your parents pay for the skiing trip you want to go on. A friend calls and tells you he has an extra ticket for a pop concert by your favourite group. The concert is on a Friday night and the tickets cost a bomb. What would you do?

Situation B

Your family are moving to a flat on the other side of the town. There is a school 5 minutes' walk away but you don't want to change schools and leave your friends. Transport will be difficult if you stay in your present school. Your younger brother will be going to the new school. What would you do?

Situation C

You are invited to a party at a friend's house. You know her/his parents are away and you are not sure who else will be there. At the last party a lot of drinking went on and things started to get out of hand. You felt very uncomfortable. What would you do?

Section 5: Safety

Activity 44: Who is responsible?

Purpose
- To show that safety is a shared responsibility
- To identify risks connected with public places

Time needed 45 minutes

What you need A set of role cards for each group of six students (see Activity Sheet 44). Enough copies of Activity Sheet 44 for each group to have one. Paper. Pens.

How you do it

1. Explain that safety is a major concern in public places. These can be areas of high or low risk according to how people behave, how regulations concerning safety are enforced, and what procedures there are for dealing with emergency situations. The class are going to look at these issues through a role play involving the Rillington Rovers Football Club.

2. Divide the class into groups of six. Give each person a card indicating which character s/he is to play at the meeting of the Rillington Rovers Football Club. The gender of the student does not have to match that of the character. Tell them to write down how they think their character would feel and react to football hooliganism.

3. Each group has 15 minutes to role play the meeting at the club and agree upon measures to deal with football hooliganism. A list of possible solutions has been suggested but the group can come up with their own. The task is to draw up a list of suggestions agreed by everyone and arranged in order of priority.

4. Each group can present their recommendations to the other groups.

5. Derole and debrief at the end of the presentations.

6. As a whole class, ask them to discuss the issues which have arisen from the role play.

Processing questions
- How did students feel during the role play?
- How were decisions made in their group?
- Is football hooliganism caused by individuals, poor facilities or attitudes of the media?
- What effects does it have on other people, the community and local environment?
- What is the difference between accidents caused by breaking rules and ignoring risks, and those caused unintentionally?
- Who makes rules and regulations concerning safety in public areas?
- Do people behave differently in a group? If 'Yes', why is this?

Section 5: Safety

Suggestions for follow-up work

- Ask students to carry out a survey of local cinemas, adventure playgrounds, leisure centres and shopping precincts. What safety regulations do they have? Are there potential dangers/risks to the public?
- Invite a local safety officer to talk to the students about their work. Use the visitor technique described in Activity 39.

SECTION 5: SAFETY

ACTIVITY SHEET 44

Rillington Rovers Football Club committee meeting

A meeting is being held at the club, at the beginning of the season, to investigate ways of reducing football hooliganism. The committee have been asked to draw up a list of recommendations. Sam Clements, the manager, has brought a list of possible solutions that he saw in the press.

Role cards

JOE BROWN – *Player*

You joined the club last season. You have a strong public following among the fans who like your aggressive play.

SAM CLEMENTS – *Football manager*

You are keen that the team gets off to a good start this season. Attendances at matches fell last year.

LIZ SIMPSON – *Secretary of the supporters' club*

You have been worried by the behaviour of some of the fans but put it down to trouble caused by visiting teams. The club wants to encourage family membership.

RONALD DART – *Police inspector*

Your force is stretched to the limit but the local community expects the police to control incidents of violence and vandalism which occur when there is a home match.

CHRIS GOODALL – *Local shopkeeper*

You lose business every time there is a home game. Your shop is near the ground and you have had to go to the expense of fitting steel shutters to protect the windows.

OBSERVER

Your task is to record what happens in the group. Do they listen to each other? What arguments do they use to support their views? How easy/difficult was it for the group to agree on their recommendations?

© A Picture of Health   Permission to photocopy this page for participant use

Section 5: Safety

Possible solutions

Improve conditions at the ground for spectators.

Prosecute players who fight on the pitch.

Suggest closing all pubs near the ground on match days.

Identify serious trouble-makers and ban them from the ground.

Make trouble-makers do Community Service on match days.

Ban visiting fans of those clubs which have caused trouble.

Encourage family membership of the supporters' club.

Section 5: Safety

Activity 45 — Keeping safe

Purpose • To help students analyse and assess situations in terms of safety

Time needed 30–40 minutes

What you need One set of situation cards (see Activity Sheet 45) for each group. Flipchart or board.

How you do it

1. Invite students to work in pairs to share their experiences of times when they have been in dangerous situations or have felt at risk. People will react to danger differently and cope in different ways. How did they feel? How were they able to cope? Encourage them to express the physical sensations – for example sweaty hands, dry throat, weak knees – and say what words describe their feelings.

2. Bring the class together and record on a flipchart or board some of their feelings when they coped well and at times when things went wrong. People can be left with feelings of hurt and anger after an event. Emphasise that it can be helpful to talk about how they felt with someone else.

3. Tell students that it can be a help to think about how to react to dangerous or risky situations in advance. Explain that they are to work with the situation cards which describe potentially dangerous situations (or they can make up scenarios of their own). Working in groups of three or four, they should choose a situation and decide what steps they would take to avoid danger/risk. Encourage them to think about the skills they would need to cope. Each group then reports back to the whole class.

4. Record the strategies suggested for each situation. Invite suggestions from groups which considered a different situation, for example being aware of risks, telling people where you are going, being able to say 'No', being able to describe emergency situations clearly on the telephone, knowing where to get help and advice.

Processing questions
- How equipped are we to cope with emergencies? Will our feelings affect the way we behave in an emergency?
- Are we able to assess potential risks/dangers?
- Is there danger in being over-confident?

Suggestions for follow-up work Get students to set up a classroom display of useful safety information, for example from the Royal Life Saving Society, the Blue Code for water safety, how to use the emergency services.

SECTION 5: SAFETY

Cards

ACTIVITY SHEET 45

Photocopy onto card and cut up before use

A friend with a motor bike offers you a lift home on the back of his bike. You have no crash helmet.

– WHAT WOULD YOU DO?
– HOW WOULD YOU FEEL?
– HOW COULD YOU AVOID IT?

On your way home from school, you think you are being followed. There are very few other people about.

– WHAT WOULD YOU DO?
– HOW WOULD YOU FEEL?
– HOW COULD YOU AVOID IT?

You are with a gang from the youth club and some have been drinking. One of them suggests a swim in the canal for a bit of a lark.

– WHAT WOULD YOU DO?
– HOW WOULD YOU FEEL?
– HOW COULD YOU AVOID IT?

You have been baby-sitting and on the way home the father tries to kiss you when he gives you a lift. He then says it was only for a laugh and asks you to keep it a secret.

– WHAT WOULD YOU DO?
– HOW WOULD YOU FEEL?
– HOW COULD YOU AVOID IT?

A group of older boys who live on the same estate invite you to come 'joy-riding' with them. You know they have been in trouble with the police but they are fun to be with.

– WHAT WOULD YOU DO?
– HOW WOULD YOU FEEL?
– HOW COULD YOU AVOID IT?

You are out on a school expedition, the countryside is unfamiliar to you and you have got separated from the rest of the group.

– WHAT WOULD YOU DO?
– HOW WOULD YOU FEEL?
– HOW COULD YOU AVOID IT?

When you are walking along with a friend, a car stops on the other side of the road. A man asks you for directions and wants you to come and show him where you are on the map.

– WHAT WOULD YOU DO?
– HOW WOULD YOU FEEL?
– HOW COULD YOU AVOID IT?

Make up one of your own.

– WHAT WOULD YOU DO?
– HOW WOULD YOU FEEL?
– HOW COULD YOU AVOID IT?

Section 5: Safety

Activity 46: Accidents do happen

Purpose
- To increase students' knowledge of the causes of accidents
- To help students to decide what to do in an emergency

Time needed   30 minutes

What you need   A copy of Activity Sheets 46A and 46B for each student. Pens.

How you do it
1. Give each student a copy of Activity Sheet 46A. Ask them to complete it individually and share their answers with a partner.
2. Bring the group together to describe the emergencies they could deal with. Give each student a copy of Activity Sheet 46B so they can check their answers.
3. Encourage them to think about those they are unsure of or would like further information about.

Processing questions
- Are students sure they know how to make an emergency call?
- Have they ever been in an emergency situation?
- How easy/difficult is it to describe a situation clearly in an emergency? Why do they think this is?

Suggestions for follow-up work
- Ask students to find out about the Blue Code of advice about water safety issued by the Royal Life Saving Society.
- Get them to make a collection of leaflets and posters concerned with safety.
- Ask them to role play in groups of three a conversation in which a person makes an emergency call to the police or fire brigade. They should take it in turns to be the caller reporting the emergency, the telephone operator and either the police or the fire brigade.

Section 5: Safety

ACTIVITY SHEET 46A

Accidents do happen!

Summary of current child accident statistics
(*Source:* Office of Population Censuses and Surveys. Adapted from 1988 figures.)

Deaths by accident type and age

Type of accident	28 days–1 yr	1–4 yrs	5–9 yrs	10–14 yrs	Total	%
Transport	12	71	136	160	379	55
Fire and flames	8	58	24	6	96	14
Suffocation	36	17	5	16	74	11
Drowning	4	29	11	4	48	7
Falls	6	11	8	10	35	5
Poisoning	1	2	0	3	6	1
Other causes	9	20	9	13	51	7
Total	76	208	193	212	689	100

KNOWLEDGE QUIZ

Do you know what to do if . . .?

	YES	NO
You are in a house by yourself when a fire breaks out	☐	☐
A small child you are looking after starts to choke	☐	☐
There is an accident in the playground and someone cuts her/himself badly	☐	☐
A friend who is a poor swimmer gets into difficulties in the water	☐	☐
You see a road accident in which a car has smashed into a bollard	☐	☐
Someone you are with burns themselves on a stove	☐	☐

© A Picture of Health   Permission to photocopy this page for participant use

Section 5: Safety

ACTIVITY SHEET 46B

Fact sheet

Fire	If there is a fire in your house, get everyone outside immediately. Do not attempt to put out the fire. Never open a door to look at a fire – this could produce a blast of flames. Dial 999 for the fire brigade. If you are trapped upstairs, get everyone together in one room away from the fire. Shut the door. Stuff sheets or blankets round the door to try to exclude the smoke. Open the windows and shout for help.
Choking	Choking occurs when someone can't breathe because their windpipe is blocked. People often splutter when food goes down the wrong way. If they are really choking, slap their back, bend them forward with their head low and slap them four times between the shoulder blades. Hold babies upside down and slap them gently. Use the Heimlich Manoeuvre if nothing else works. To do this, get behind the person and put your arms around her/his middle. Make a fist with one hand and grasp it with the other. Pull sharply inwards and upwards. Repeat this four times together with back slapping. Dial 999 for an ambulance.
Cuts and bleeding	Press on the cut with your fingers or whole hand. Keep the pressure on until the blood flow stops – for 5 to 15 minutes. Never apply a tourniquet; pressure from the hand is enough. If there is an object in a wound, leave it there and apply a light dressing over the area. If the injury is to the arm or leg, raise the limb to reduce the blood flow. Dial 999 and ask for an ambulance.
Swimmer in difficulty	Do not go into the water. Look for something such as a broom to help pull the person out. Throw in any floating objects available for them to hold on to. Call 999 and ask for the police or the coastguard service.
Road accident (car)	Never move injured people unless you have to. Be reassuring to those involved and keep them warm. Drivers should try to warn other motorists in order to prevent more vehicles crashing and should check that their ignition is switched off. If someone is unconscious it is most important to check their airway (throat and windpipe) is clear. Never remove helmets from injured motor cyclists.

© A Picture of Health   Permission to photocopy this page for participant use

Section 5: Safety

Burns and scalds

Immerse the burnt area under cold water at once and keep there for at least 10 minutes. Burns become more serious unless they are cooled quickly. It is important that no ointments or powders, or butter or flour, are applied to a burn. Lessen shock by reassuring the person and loosen their clothing, but NOT if it is stuck to the skin. If burns are severe the injured person must go to hospital. Dial 999 for an ambulance.

NB People often think that someone else has dialled 999 in an emergency when in fact no one has. Always check.

SECTION 5: SAFETY

ACTIVITY 47 — *Bullying*

Purpose • To help students think about how to deal with incidents of bullying

Time 30 minutes

What you need Copies of Activity Sheets 47A and 47B for each student. Pens.

How you do it
1. Divide the class into small groups to discuss what the outcomes of each situation on Activity Sheet 47A might be and what they could do to help or advise in each situation.
2. Bring the groups together to report back and consider any differences in what is suggested.
3. Re-form the students into small groups. Ask them to think about what sort of people are likely to bully others. Get them to look at the list on Activity Sheet 47B and pick out people they think are likely to be bullies.
4. Bring the class together to compare answers.

Processing questions
- What sort of people bully others?
- Is there such a thing as a typical bully?
- Bullying can be mental as well as physical. Can the class think of examples of mental bullying?
- Is there a difference between teasing and bullying?
- Are certain types of people likely to get bullied and, if so, why?

Suggestions for follow-up work
- Ask students to write a story which features a young person being bullied and how they coped with it.
- Get the class to draw up a code of behaviour which would help reduce bullying. Ask them to discuss how it could be put into practice.

SECTION 5: SAFETY

ACTIVITY SHEET 47A

Bullying

SCENARIOS

Two friends are crossing the park on the way to school when they see a group of older boys walking towards them.

How would the friends feel? Why? What might they do?

Ben is 14. All his friends are taller than he is. They tease him about his size and he is self-conscious about his looks. He has just been told he has to start wearing glasses.

What can Ben do about the behaviour of his friends?

Is there anything he can do for himself? What should his friends do? Share your ideas.

Two students are on their own in the cloakroom.

    A: 'Give me some cash to get some lunch. I've left mine at home.'
    B: 'Sorry, I can't – I need it to get home.'
    A: 'Right! I'll get you after school – just you watch out.'

B doesn't like A and is worried that the threat will be carried out. Discuss what you think might happen. Is there a sensible way of dealing with the situation? What advice would you give to the person being threatened? Have you ever been in a similar situation? What did you do?

You come across one of the first-year students near the bicycle sheds. S/he seems very distressed. You see someone from your class walking away laughing with a can of Coke in their hand. You think they have taken it from the first-year. What could you do?

© A Picture of Health   Permission to photocopy this page for participant use

SECTION 5: SAFETY

ACTIVITY SHEET 47B

Bullying

WHO ARE THE BULLIES?

Read the list and tick those people you think are most likely to be bullies. Why do you think this is?

- [ ] 1 Someone who is very clever
- [ ] 2 Someone who is always telling tales
- [ ] 3 Someone who is good at games
- [ ] 4 Someone who is no good at games
- [ ] 5 Someone who feels unsure of herself or himself
- [ ] 6 Someone who can stand up for herself or himself
- [ ] 7 Someone who is a loner
- [ ] 8 Someone who has a lot of friends
- [ ] 9 Someone who is bossy
- [ ] 10 Someone who thinks they know everything
- [ ] 11 Someone who will not share
- [ ] 12 Someone who enjoys a laugh
- [ ] 13 Someone who flies into a temper easily
- [ ] 14 Someone whose parents are very rich
- [ ] 15 Someone who is bigheaded

Complete one of your own

- [ ]   Someone who is . . .

Section 5: Safety

Activity 48: *Vandalism*

Purpose
- To explore perceptions of vandalism

Time 30 minutes

What you need Newspaper articles, drawings, illustrations, photographs – ask students to bring in anything which they think shows an aspect of vandalism (pollution of the environment, damage to property). Sheets of flipchart paper with lines to look like a brick wall, cut into four jigsaw pieces. Felt tip pens. Optional resource Activity Sheet 48.

How you do it
1. Working in groups of four, invite students to choose one of the items collected and discuss their reaction to it. Appoint a person to report back, describing their piece of material and what they thought about it. What connection did they think the material had with vandalism?
2. Give each student a piece of a brick wall jigsaw and ask them to draw and/or write what the word VANDALISM means to them. Ask them, in groups of four, to complete their jigsaw and talk through their drawings. Display the jigsaws. Get them to discuss whether there are similarities between their perceptions of vandalism; whether some kinds of vandalism are worse than others; what makes them worse; and if there is such a thing as a typical vandal. If appropriate compare the students' perceptions with the definitions of vandalism on Activity Sheet 48.
3. Divide students into different groups of four. Invite them to discuss the following:
   - How vandalism features in their lives – in school and home and outside in the community.
   - Whether there are opportunities to do something about vandalism.
   - What they would like done about it. Encourage students to specify ideas.
4. Each group then prepares a report to present to the whole class.

Suggestions for follow-up work
- Encourage students to find out about any examples of ways in which vandalism has been reduced in either their school or neighbourhood.
- Suggest they make up a play which illustrates the effect of vandalism on a person whose property has been damaged.
- This activity links with Activity 20 in Section 2.

SECTION 5: SAFETY

Vandalism

ACTIVITY SHEET 48

FACT SHEET

Vandalism – Criminal damage

In Great Britain, the term 'vandalism' does not appear in the criminal law. The vandal is usually dealt with under Section 1(1) of the Criminal Damage Act 1971. This says that criminal damage occurs when:

Anyone who without lawful authority . . .
1. destroys or damages any property belonging to another, or
2. intends to destroy or damage such property, or
3. is so reckless in his/her actions, as to whether or not such property is damaged, he/she is guilty of an offence which may be subject to a fine or term of imprisonment.

Other crimes which might be interpreted as acts of vandalism could be dealt with under other sections of the criminal law, for example the Litter Act 1982.

Six different kinds of vandalism

(Adapted from an essay on property destruction, motives and meaning by Professor Stanley Cohen, published in *Vandalism*, edited by Colin Ward, Architectural Press, 1973.)

1. **Acquisitive vandalism**
   Breaking open telephone coin boxes, electricity or gas meters, slot machines; stripping lead and wire from buildings etc.

2. **Tactical vandalism**
   Breaking a window in order to be arrested and get a bed for the night in prison; jamming a machine in a factory to enforce a rest period or draw attention to a complaint.

3. **Ideological vandalism**
   Like tactical vandalism, but intended to further an ideological cause or campaign, or to put over a message, eg painting slogans on walls, breaking embassy windows in a demonstration.

Section 5: Safety

4 **Vindictive vandalism**
For example, breaking the windows of a youth club or school to settle a grudge against the club leader or headteacher.

5 **Play vandalism**
Destruction in the course of a game; eg who can break the most windows in an empty house or shoot out the most street lights.

6 **Malicious vandalism**
This is often directed at public property and seems to be an expression of rage or frustration. Cohen associates it with feelings of boredom, despair, exasperation, resentment and failure.

SECTION 6

Substance use and misuse

SECTION 6: SUBSTANCE USE AND MISUSE

ACTIVITY 49
Alphabetical brainstorm

Purpose
- To explore students' existing knowledge about drugs
- To stimulate further discussion about drugs

Time needed 30 minutes

What you need Large sheets of paper and pens

How you do it
1. Point out that, as they live in a drug-taking society, all of them will have some experience and knowledge concerning drugs – it may be knowing someone who smokes, taking an aspirin, having a glass of 'bubbly' at a wedding. Explain the purpose of the activity.
2. With students working in groups of four, ask each group to write the letters of the alphabet down the left-hand side of a large sheet of paper. For each letter, they are to think of as many words as they can connected with drugs and drug-taking; for example H might suggest hangover, heroin, hash, happiness, hopelessness. (Depending on the time available, the groups could work on all or some of the letters.)
3. Bring the groups back together to share results.

Processing questions
- Which drugs have they named – are they mainly legal or illegal?
- How many words were street or slang terms?
- How many were connected with the effects of drug-taking and were those positive or negative?
- Were there any words describing how a drug is taken?
- Is there any further information that they would like?

Suggestions for follow-up work Activities to give more information, such as Activity 50 and Activity 53.

SECTION 6: SUBSTANCE USE AND MISUSE

ACTIVITY 50: Types of drugs

Purpose	• To provide information about different types of drugs
Time needed	20 minutes
What you need	Copies of Activity Sheets 50A and 50B for each student. Pens.
How you do it	1 Give each student a copy of Activity Sheet 50A and ask them to match each definition in Column A with the correct word in Column B. 2 Get them to share their answers with a partner. Ask them to think about whether there are any differences in their responses. 3 Hand out Activity Sheet 50B and go through the answers.
Processing questions	• Did they have difficulty with any of the words? • Did any of the answers surprise them? • Are there any other drugs (or expressions) which they have heard about and do not understand?
Suggestions for follow-up work	If students need more information, contact an organisation specialising in drug use and abuse, such as ISDD or TACADE (addresses on page 229), or your local health promotion unit. They may be able to supply you with leaflets and articles appropriate for the age group. Follow the method described in Activity 32, from step 2 using 'drugs' as the focus rather than 'contraception' for step 5. Give out the leaflets which you have acquired.

SECTION 6: SUBSTANCE USE AND MISUSE

Types of drugs

ACTIVITY SHEET 50A

Drugs are non-food substances that can affect the way your mind and body work. The immediate effects of taking a drug will depend on the **type** of drug, the **amount** taken, the **mood** the person is in when s/he takes it, and the **situation** in which the drug is taken.

You should know as much as you can about drugs that are available, both legally and illegally. You need to have accurate information about their uses and the harmful effects of misuse or abuse. That will mean that you will be able to make responsible decisions about using drugs.

Find out how much you know by matching each definition in Column A with the correct word in Column B.

Column A

a) drugs that slow down the nervous system

b) a stimulant found in coffee, tea and some pills sold over the counter

c) drugs that excite the nervous system

d) any drug, such as marijuana, that is prepared from the hemp plant

e) drugs that relieve pain

f) drugs that cause people to hear or see things differently or abnormally

g) inhaled vapours that are absorbed through the lungs and rapidly reach the brain

h) drugs that are used to increase muscle bulk and strength

i) a chemical found in tobacco

j) stimulants used to 'speed' performance

Column B

1 caffeine

2 depressants

3 hallucinogens

4 solvents

5 amphetamines

6 opiates

7 cannabis

8 stimulants

9 anabolic steroids

10 nicotine

SECTION 6: SUBSTANCE USE AND MISUSE

ACTIVITY SHEET 50B

Answers

a) 2: Depressants slow down the body systems and the functioning of the brain. They relax, tranquillise and make people sleepy. People who have taken a mild depressant often feel less inhibited. Drugs of this type include alcohol, tranquillisers and barbiturates.

b) 1: Caffeine is a mild stimulant. A cup of instant coffee contains about 65mg of caffeine, tea 60mg, a can of soft drink 30–50mg and some of the best-known brands of analgesics or pain-killers contain up to 50mg in each tablet.

c) 8: Stimulants speed up the action of the brain. They make people feel more alert and confident and less tired. Large doses can make a person feel confused and agitated, and may cause high blood pressure and irregular heartbeat. Drugs of this type include amphetamines ('speed'), caffeine, cocaine, crack and tobacco.

d) 7: Hashish or hash, the commonest form of cannabis in the UK, is resin scraped or rubbed from the plant and pressed into blocks. It is usually smoked as a cigarette or 'joint'.

e) 6: Opiates relieve pain, create a feeling of detachment, and in large doses produce a 'high'. Examples are opium, heroin and morphine.

f) 3: These are sometimes called psychedelic or mind-altering drugs. They include LSD, hallucinogenic ('magic') mushrooms and ecstasy.

g) 4: Sniffing solvents (including glue sniffing) produces effects similar to drinking alcohol. Repeated or deep sniffing can cause an 'overdose', loss of control and unconsciousness.

h) 9: Anabolic steroids include chemicals which relate to the male hormone testosterone. They are sometimes misused in sport to improve performance. In teenagers who have not fully developed, they can stunt growth. Long-term use can cause severe physical problems.

i) 10: Tobacco contains a variety of chemicals. These include nicotine, a mild stimulant found naturally only in tobacco leaves.

j) 5: Amphetamines, sometimes called 'speed' or 'pep pills', are used to treat some disorders of the nervous system. They are also taken illegally, to make people feel more confident and cheerful and help them to stay awake. They produce an increase in energy and alertness. They may also raise the heart rate and blood pressure.

SECTION 6: SUBSTANCE USE AND MISUSE

Activity 51: *Is it OK?*

Purpose	• To examine attitudes to drug use • To consider the social acceptability of various drugs
Time needed	20 minutes
What you need	Cards, A4 size, each with the name of a drug on it in large letters: AMPHETAMINES, ALCOHOL, ASPIRIN, CAFFEINE, CANNABIS, CIGARETTES, COCAINE, ECSTASY, HEROIN, MORPHINE, PARA-CETAMOL, SOLVENTS, TRANQUILLISERS. A space large enough for everyone to stand in a line.
How you do it	1 Ask each student to take a card at random. Make sure they have all heard of the drug on their card. 2 Ask them to imagine they are 20+ years old. Would it be OK for them to take the drug whose name they are holding? Get them to imagine a line within the room, with 'VERY OK' at one end and 'NOT AT ALL OK' at the other. Tell them to position themselves along that line, holding their cards for others to see. 3 Ask the students to turn to the person next to them and share why they are standing there. 4 Point out that they can change position if they want. Ask them to consider whether anything would make a difference to the position (eg the amount of drug taken, the frequency, what you have to do after taking it)? Is there anyone else in the line who they think should move? If so, they should try to persuade them to change position.
Processing questions	• Which drugs are considered acceptable in society? Do they know of any other countries where or times when this was different? • Are there different reasons for using drugs? • Do they think some reasons are more acceptable than others?
Suggestions for follow-up work	Social acceptability could be explored further by considering the laws relating to drug use, as analysed in Activity Sheet 51. More detailed information is available from ISDD (for address see page 230).

SECTION 6: SUBSTANCE USE AND MISUSE

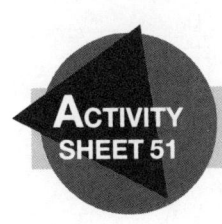

Drugs and the law

ACTIVITY SHEET 51

Drug	Buying/ possessing	Being intoxicated	Supplying
Alcohol	Illegal to buy if under 18 (but from 16 you may buy beer or cider with meal)	Illegal to be drunk in a public place Illegal to drive over the limit	Illegal to *sell* to under-18s (except beer or cider with a meal to 16s and 17s) Illegal to *give* to under-5s
Tobacco	No offence	No offence	Illegal to *sell* to under-16s
Solvents	No offence	No offence Breach of peace if sniffing in public place Illegal to drive while unfit to do so through drugs	Illegal if suspected to be sniffed by a person under 18
Magic mushrooms	No offence unless prepared (eg cooked)	No offence Illegal to drive while unfit to do so through drugs	No offence unless prepared
Tranquillisers	No offence	As above	Illegal, unless on prescription

Heroin
Cocaine
Amphetamines
LSD
Ecstasy
Barbiturates
Cannabis
Opium

} All illegal to supply, buy or possess. No offence to be intoxicated, although illegal to drive while unfit to do so through drugs.

151 © A Picture of Health   Permission to photocopy this page for participant use

Section 6: Substance Use and Misuse

Activity 52: Why do people take drugs?

Purpose
- To explore why some people take drugs
- To discuss stereotypes of drug-users

Time needed 30–40 minutes

What you need A set of people cards (see Activity Sheet 52). Large sheets of paper. Felt-tip pens.

How you do it

1. Working in small groups of three or four, give each group one of the people cards on Activity Sheet 52.
2. Ask the groups to think about a typical weekday and weekend for the person on their card. What types of drug might that person take? Each group should list the drugs and then, for each drug, jot down the reasons why the person might take it.
3. In the whole group, ask them to call out drugs that they have identified. Write each one on the top of a separate sheet of paper and display the sheets round the walls. Appoint a scribe for each sheet.
4. For each drug, ask the groups if they had written down that it might be taken by the person on their card. The scribe should jot down the characteristics of the people concerned.
5. Next, collect the reasons written down for taking a particular drug and again ask the scribe to jot these on the relevant sheet.
6. Discuss the results in the whole group.

Processing questions
- Which drugs were frequently mentioned? Why might this be? Is it because they are legal and socially acceptable, or are they 'flavour of the month' and so on everybody's mind?
- Are certain drugs associated with certain types of people? What are the dangers of stereotyping people and drug-users in this way?
- Are there any similarities in the reasons given for taking the different drugs? Can the reasons be grouped in any way? Can they think of any other reasons which did not come from thinking about the people on the cards?
- What do they think are the main reasons for people their age using drugs (eg cigarettes, alcohol, solvents)?

Suggestions for follow-up work Working in small groups, ask students to choose one of the reasons and discuss what a person could do instead of taking drugs.

SECTION 6: SUBSTANCE USE AND MISUSE

ACTIVITY SHEET 52

People cards

Photocopy on to card and cut up before use.

Man, 17. Doing a course in engineering at further education college. Plays in a reggae band. Lives in a large terraced house with his parents, two sisters and an older brother. Spends most evenings out with his friends.

Woman, 18. At sixth-form college, taking three A-levels. Lives at home in a detached, expensive house. Father is a company director. Has her own car, a Beetle. Holidays abroad with friends. Goes to nightclubs and discos. Works as a waitress at the weekend. Boyfriend is at university.

Woman, 35. Single parent with 7-year-old child. Divorced. Social worker. Lives in a small Victorian semi-detached house. Finds her job stressful. Practises yoga. Vegetarian.

Woman, 28. Full-time housewife with two young children. Lives on a small estate of modern, up-market houses in north-east. Husband is 30 and a computer programmer. Suffering from depression.

Man, 45. Married. Unemployed. Was a bricklayer with a large building firm. Two children – 17-year-old daughter at further education college, 14-year-old son at school. Wife also unemployed. Receiving unemployment pay and income support. Lives in council house which they are buying. Goes to the pub at lunchtimes and on several evenings a week.

Man, 21. In his final year, studying philosophy and psychology at university. Lives on campus, in a students' hall of residence. Works in a pub two evenings a week and some weekends. Wants to travel when he has finished his studies, particularly to India.

SECTION 6: SUBSTANCE USE AND MISUSE

Girl, 15. At school. Bright. Expected to do well in GCSE. Likes pop music and going to discos. Sometimes goes to the pub with friends. Earns £16 from a Saturday job. Father works as a car mechanic and mother teaches shorthand and typing at local college.

Boy, 12. At school. Often plays truant. Good at sport, especially football. Finds academic subjects difficult. Lives with his mother and older brother. Has a paper round. Pocket money of £2 per week. Meets his friends most evenings on some waste ground.

Woman, 46. Married. Both children, aged 22 and 20, have left home. The 20-year-old daughter is at university. Husband is a 50-year-old dentist. Lives in a detached house in Hampshire. Belongs to a golf and country club. Teaches English part-time.

Woman, 77. Widowed for five years. Lives alone in a council flat. Daughter lives nearby. Pension is only income. Suffers from breathlessness, blocked arteries and coughing fits, especially in the morning. Member of the Women's Institute.

Man, 28. Single. Works in marketing for a large company. Has his own flat in Surrey. Usually has lunch in pub. During the week he often does not get home from work until 8 or 9pm. Enjoys parties and going out 'with the lads' at weekends. Worried that he is putting on weight.

SECTION 6: SUBSTANCE USE AND MISUSE

ACTIVITY 53: The effects of drugs

Purpose • To provide information about the effects of drug-taking

Time needed 30 minutes

What you need A copy of Activity Sheet 53 for each student. Pens.

How you do it
1. Hand out Activity Sheet 53 and inform students that this is a guide for them, not a test to be passed or failed.
2. Ask them to put their answers, TRUE or FALSE, in the spaces provided.
3. When everyone has finished, read out the answers, allowing students to correct their own papers.
4. Discuss answers.

Processing questions
- For which questions were they most sure of the answers?
- Why was that? Where had they got that information from?
- Were there any answers that surprised them?
- Is there anything they would like to know more about?

Suggestions for follow-up work Divide the class into small groups. Give each group a card on which is written the name of a different drug, one which could be used by their age group (eg alcohol, cigarettes, cannabis, solvents). Ask each group to draw a person and to write around that person all the possible effects of taking that drug – short term, long term, physical and social. Hand out fact sheets about the drugs (available from organisations such as ISDD and TACADE; for addresses see page 229). Check accuracy of groupwork.

Answers for Activity Sheet 53

1. True
2. True; depends on, eg, where you are, who you are with, the mood you're in and what you expect to happen
3. False; reactions can be slower than normal – both mental and physical
4. False
5. True
6. False
7. True
8. True
9. True
10. True
11. False

Section 6: Substance Use and Misuse

The effects of drugs

Activity Sheet 53

Mark the following statements true or false

	TRUE	FALSE
1 Young people are more easily affected by alcohol than those over 20.		
2 The same drug can affect you differently at different times.		
3 Cannabis is safer than drink for drivers.		
4 You can do everything better after a couple of drinks		
5 Allowing people to use illegal drugs in your house could lead to prosecution.		
6 Coffee or a cold shower sobers you up.		
7 Up to 100,000 people die each year in the UK as a result of cigarette smoking.		
8 Sniffing solvents has a similar effect to taking alcoholic drinks.		
9 People who drink a lot of coffee and then stop suddenly can get headaches.		
10 If someone stops taking ecstasy, they can feel tired and depressed for several days.		
11 However much alcohol you drink on one occasion, you cannot kill yourself.		

SECTION 6: SUBSTANCE USE AND MISUSE

ACTIVITY 54

Carousel

Purpose
- To identify what makes it easy or difficult to refuse drugs
- To practise saying 'No'

Time needed 20–30 minutes

What you need A room arranged so that people can sit in pairs and the pairs can then rotate round, changing partners. Ideally this means two concentric circles, but this may not be possible in your classroom setting.

How you do it
1. Ask for suggestions of situations in which a person might be offered a drug, and feel it was difficult to refuse. Remind them that alcohol and cigarettes are drugs.
2. Ask them to sit in pairs, preferably facing one another as in the illustration. Call those in the inner circle (or on the left-hand side if they are sitting in pairs in rows) A, and those in the outer circle (or on the right-hand side) B.
3. Choose a scenario – preferably from situations mentioned by students, but failing that from the list below.
   - Someone who has been hanging around after school offers to sell you some 'uppers' for a couple of £s.
   - Someone you know is having a party while their parents are away. They say you're welcome, as long as you bring a bottle of something alcoholic.
   - You are out one evening with someone you think is great fun. He says he's got hold of something special and takes out a joint. He offers you a smoke.
   - A friend comes round to your house. In your room s/he is about to light a cigarette. Your parents don't allow smoking in the house.
4. Ask A to be the persuader and B to resist. Keep things snappy – 2 minutes will probably be long enough. Ask them to share how they felt during this. Did they both end up feeling OK? Did anyone get in their way, leaving the other feeling bad?
5. Choose another scenario. Rotate one circle (or row), changing partners so that the As meet a different B. This time B is to be the persuader and A is to resist. Afterwards ask them to share how it felt.
6. Repeat steps 4 and 5 with new partners and scenarios.
7. Combine the final pairs to form groups of four students. Ask them to discuss which situation they found most difficult and why. Did they come up with anything which seemed to help in resisting pressure?
8. Hold a plenary discussion to draw out the learning.

SECTION 6: SUBSTANCE USE AND MISUSE

Processing questions
- Was there anything which seemed effective in resisting pressure?
- Does it make any difference who they are with, or how many people there are around?
- What else will affect how they behave?

Suggestions for follow-up work
- Divide the class into small groups. Ask each group to think of a situation involving someone of their age and either legal or illegal drugs. Get them to write this on an index card and pass it on to the next group. They are to consider what the person would need to be able to do (what skills?), how they would need to feel and what they would need to know (what information?) to be able to cope. Ask the whole group to share their responses.
- Activities 9 and 10 on assertiveness. Activity Sheet 9 may be useful in discussing their responses in the carousel exercise.

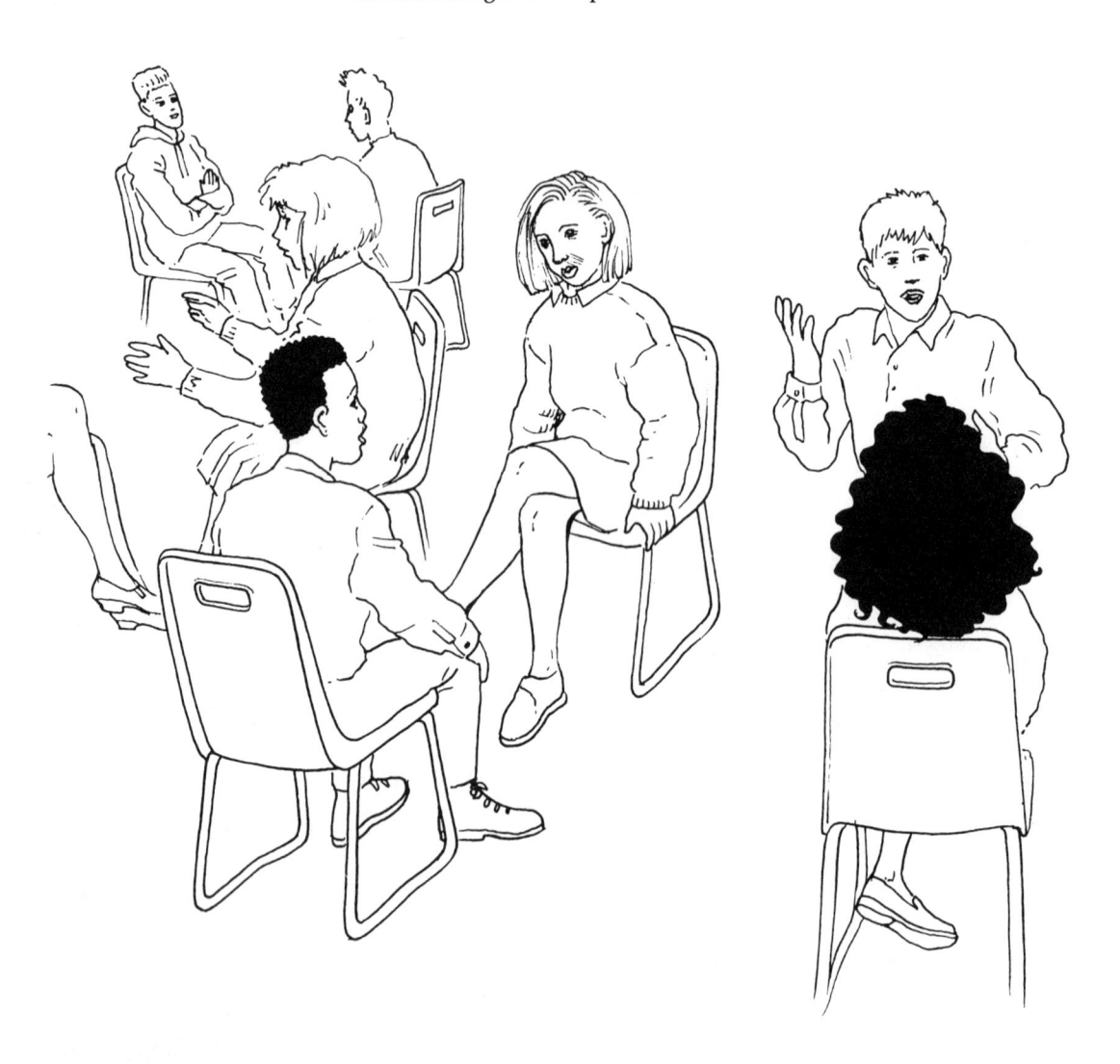

Section 6: Substance Use and Misuse

Activity 55

Do you know what you're taking?

Purpose
- To provide information about the amount of alcohol in different drinks
- To discuss the difficulty in calculating what and how much of a drug students might be taking

Time needed 20 minutes

What you need A copy of Activity Sheet 55 for each student. Calculators. Pens.

How you do it
1. Give each student a copy of Activity Sheet 55. Ask them to solve the puzzle. Work through the first example, a can of lager, with them to make sure they know how to do it.
2. Read out the answers and encourage discussion.

Processing questions
- Were they surprised by any of the results?
- When would it be most difficult for people to work out how much alcohol they were drinking?
- What do they think of people who lace others' drinks or make very strong punch?
- If it is difficult to tell exactly what you are taking with alcohol, how about other drugs? Do people always know what they are buying?
- What are the dangers of mixing drugs, for example alcohol and pain-killers?

Suggestions for follow-up work
- Ask groups to carry out research in supermarkets into the alcoholic content by volume of different drinks. Beer, for example, can be from 3% to 10%.
- Ask them to concoct an interesting non-alcoholic drink.

Answer for Activity Sheet 55

The pint of beer contains the most alcohol.

SECTION 6: SUBSTANCE USE AND MISUSE

ACTIVITY SHEET 55

Do you know what you are taking?

Can you solve the following puzzle? Someone you know is having a party and has bought a range of drinks at the supermarket. Bottles and cans now show the amount of alcohol in them as percentages of alcohol per volume (where this is above 1.2%), so that people can compare strengths.

The bottles, cans and glasses are all set out on a table. Some of them are listed below.

Which contains the most alcohol?

For each drink, in the first column write down the size of the drink in ml. You will find all the information you need on this activity sheet.

To find out how much alcohol the drink contains, using a calculator, multiply the figure in the first column by the alcoholic content by volume (the figure in the second column). Write your answer in the third column.

Information to help you

There are 7 wine glasses in a 75cl bottle of wine
There are 12 sherry glasses in a 70cl bottle of sherry
1 gill = ¼ pint
1 can = 440ml or roughly ¾ pint

	1 Total number of ml	2 Alcoholic content by volume	3 ml of alcohol
A can of lager	440ml	3.4%	14.96ml
A glass of wine		12%	
A bottle of low-alcohol lager	330ml	0.05%	
A pub measure of whisky (⅙ gill)		40%	
A pint of beer		4%	
A can of cider		3%	
A glass of sherry		17.5%	

160 © A Picture of Health   Permission to photocopy this page for participant use

Section 6: Substance Use and Misuse

Measures at home or at parties may not be the same as pub measures.

The same type of drink can vary enormously in strength. Did you know that extra strength cider contains almost three times as much alcohol as ordinary cider?

As a guide, the following drinks all contain roughly the same amount of alcohol, about 10ml (known as 1 unit):

> 1 unit = ½ pint of beer = 1 glass of wine = 1 measure of spirits = 1 small sherry

If you have an alcoholic drink, your blood alcohol level increases. On average it takes an hour for the body to get rid of 1 unit (10ml) of alcohol. It can be dangerous to drink too much in one session.

SECTION 6: SUBSTANCE USE AND MISUSE

ACTIVITY 56
Anti-smoking

Purpose
- To get reactions to anti-smoking materials
- To consider measures which might be effective in discouraging smoking

Time needed 30 minutes

What you need A collection of anti-smoking posters (from your local health promotion unit) displayed around the walls. Pin a sheet of paper next to each. A few advertisements for cigarettes. Pens.

How you do it

1. Explain that although it has been proved that smoking can lead to serious illness and death, recent surveys suggest that one in ten children between 11 and 15 is still a regular smoker. Point out that £100 million a year is spent by the tobacco industry in promoting its products. Show examples of advertisements and discuss some of the techniques used.

2. Organisations such as the Health Education Authority have only £2.2 million from the Department of Health for anti-smoking work. Ask the students to wander round and look at the posters on the walls, choosing two which they like for some reason. They should put their name on the sheet of paper next to the posters they choose.

3. Ask each student to find someone who likes the same poster as her/himself and talk together about why they like it. You may have to pair a few students who have made different choices.

4. In the whole group, ask them to share the reasons for choosing posters.

Processing questions
- What do they like about any of the posters?
- Which posters had no names next to them? Why might this be?
- Are different things likely to appeal to different people/age groups?
- How successful do they think the posters are in discouraging smoking?
- What other measures should be carried out to combat the large sums of money spent on advertising by tobacco companies?
- Activity 18 looks at techniques used by advertisers to promote products.

Suggestions for follow-up work Ask each student to design an anti-smoking poster for display in the school, possibly in conjunction with National No Smoking Day.

SECTION 7

Food and nutrition

Section 7: Food and Nutrition

Activity 57: A healthy appetite

Purpose
- To check students' knowledge of good nutrition and its importance for health
- To produce a guide to healthy eating

Time needed 30 minutes

What you need A copy of Activity Sheet 57A for each student. Pens.

How you do it
1. Give each student a copy of Activity Sheet 57A. Ask them to work in pairs.
2. Explain that the quiz is a way for them to check their knowledge of what is meant by healthy eating.
3. Divide them into pairs. Ask them to answer the questions in the space provided.
4. When everyone has finished, get them to discuss each statement. Read out the correct answers from Activity Sheet 57B.
5. Encourage a discussion on healthy eating in the whole group.

Processing questions
- How accurate was their information about healthy eating?
- Where has their knowledge come from? Is it parents, TV programmes, health promotion leaflets and advertising, newspaper articles?
- Did any of the answers surprise them?
- Does knowing about healthy eating make any difference to their own diet?
- How many students eat breakfast? What reasons do people give for not eating breakfast? Can they suggest easy nutritious breakfast choices?

Suggestions for follow-up work A personal survey – ask the students to keep a record for a week and find out the ten foods they eat most often. They should then draw a chart and put ticks in the appropriate column showing:

FA = Food high in fat
FI = Food high in fibre
SU = Food high in sugar
SA = Food high in salt
NU = Food that is a nutritious snack
NNU = Food that is not nutritious

Get them to share the information with the rest of the class after a week.

SECTION 7: FOOD AND NUTRITION

ACTIVITY SHEET 57A

Food quiz

		TRUE	FALSE
1	Potatoes are fattening	☐	☐
2	You can be healthy on a diet without meat	☐	☐
3	Bread and pasta are fattening	☐	☐
4	Good nutrition will protect you from illness in the future	☐	☐
5	Going without breakfast does no harm	☐	☐
6	Fat is an essential part of our diet	☐	☐
7	If you have a healthy diet, you will get all the vitamins you need	☐	☐
8	A glass of an ordinary soft drink contains five teaspoons of sugar	☐	☐
9	Half the sugar we eat is hidden in other foods	☐	☐
10	Steak is more nutritious than chicken	☐	☐
11	Fibre-rich foods are important for good health	☐	☐
12	Most people don't need to worry about the amount of salt they eat	☐	☐

SECTION 7: FOOD AND NUTRITION

ACTIVITY SHEET 57B

Answer sheet

1 FALSE Potatoes alone are not fattening. They are a healthy food, high in fibre, and if you eat the skin they provide you with vitamins. They *are* fattening when fried, eaten as crisps, filled with butter or roasted.

2 TRUE Some people choose to exclude all meat from their diets. These people are VEGETARIANS. There are different types; some eat fish and other animal products, whilst others exclude all meat, fish and poultry. Some simply avoid red meats. VEGANS are people who consume no foods of animal origin. Their diets are made up of vegetables, vegetable oils, cereals, nuts, fruits and seeds. Whether or not a vegetarian diet is adequate nutritionally will depend on the range and amounts of food eaten.

3 FALSE These foods, especially wholemeal varieties, are low in fats. They fill you up without giving too many calories – useful if you are watching your weight. Remember it's not the bread that makes you fat, but what you spread on it! Foods naturally rich in fibre have lots of vitamins and other nutrients too. Fibre is not lost in cooking. Fibre helps your intestines to eliminate waste products easily, therefore preventing constipation. It is also a good protection against cancer of the colon (large intestine).

4 TRUE Healthy eating habits are important to teenagers; their bodies are growing and changing rapidly. A nutritious diet helps prevent diseases such as heart disease, certain forms of cancer and obesity. Vitamins and minerals found in food control the work of other nutrients in the body. If you have a healthy diet, you will get all the vitamins you need from the food you eat.

5 FALSE Without breakfast a person may soon feel physically and mentally exhausted. If they have not eaten for 12 hours, their blood sugar level drops and they may feel lethargic and find it difficult to concentrate.

6 TRUE Fats are a concentrated source of energy and they provide the body with heat: 1g of fat provides twice as much food energy as 1g of carbohydrate. However, in the UK we tend to eat too much fat, and this can lead to being overweight. There are two different sorts of fat:

SATURATED FATS – found in animal fats (beef, lamb, pork, suet, lard) and dairy products (milk, cheese, butter); also in some vegetable fats (eg palm oil) and in chocolates, hard margarines, sauces, puddings. Certain types of saturated fats are linked to a higher risk of heart disease. The more saturated fat you eat, the more cholesterol there will be in

Section 7: Food and Nutrition

your blood. This builds up, blocking arteries and perhaps causing a heart attack.
POLYUNSATURATES – in vegetable oils (like sunflower, soya, corn oil), soft margarine, nuts, oily fish. They do not raise cholesterol in the same way as saturated fats do. They help make and repair body cells.

For healthy eating, try to cut down the total amount of fat you eat.

7 TRUE   If you have a healthy diet you will get all the vitamins you need from the food you eat (eg a small glass of orange juice supplies all the vitamin C you need in a day). Some vitamins can be stored in the body (vitamins A, D, E, K). An intake of vitamins B and C is needed each day.

8 TRUE   When buying soft drinks choose low-calorie ones or unsweetened fruit juices diluted with water. Sugar gives you 'empty calories', that is calories with no other nutrients – no vitamins, no minerals, no fibre, no protein. Eating too much sugar causes tooth decay and makes you fat.

9 TRUE   In Britain, on average we buy 1lb of sugar a week. We eat *twice* that amount because of all the sugar contained in processed food – sweets, drinks, biscuits, cakes. Labels showing names such as SUCROSE, GLUCOSE, DEXTROSE, FRUCTOSE and MALTOSE indicate sugars. They are found in soups, sauces and even savoury biscuits. They all help to make you fat.

10 FALSE   Red meat such as steak is a good source of iron, but many foods provide iron – examples are bread and cereals, pulses and green vegetables. Steak provides us with protein and vitamins, but chicken is equally good. Cheaper lean cuts of meat are just as nutritious as expensive ones. It's better to grill than to fry food. Casseroling and stewing are good ways to cook meats.

11 TRUE   Fibre is the name given to a special group of carbohydrates. Fibre comes from beans, brown rice, wholemeal pasta, vegetables and brown bread. You don't get any fibre in animal products such as cheese, eggs and meat. Fibre-rich foods fill you up without giving too many calories. They may protect against bowel problems, including cancer of the bowel, which is one of the commonest forms of cancer in Britain.

12 FALSE   On average we eat 10g of salt a day – two whole teaspoonfuls. Everyone needs some salt, but most people don't need more than 1g a day! For some people eating too much salt can contribute to high blood pressure, which in turn can cause heart disease and strokes. More than half the salt we eat is added by manufacturers who process our food. It's a good idea to cut down on salty snack foods like crisps and salted nuts. Remember there is a lot of salt in bacon and ham.

Section 7: Food and Nutrition

Activity 58 — Diet and lifestyles

Purpose
- To help students understand the link between diet and lifestyle
- To make students aware of the problems of hunger and food shortage in some countries

Time needed 30 minutes

What you need A set of menu cards and country cards (from Activity Sheet 58) for each group. Complete copies of Activity Sheet 58, one per student.

How you do it
1. Explain that 'diet' means what we eat over a period of time to meet our needs for food. Our diet is affected by our 'lifestyle' or the way in which we live. Invite students to suggest how they think people's lifestyles have changed during this century. Record the suggestions. Ask if some lifestyles are healthier than others, and whether the class can offer reasons.
2. Point out that different people will have different lifestyles which will vary according to where they live. Divide students into small groups and give each group a set of menu cards and country cards. Can they match the menu to the country?
3. Bring the groups together to check their answers. Hand out a complete copy of Activity Sheet 58, as an answer sheet, to each student.

Processing questions
- Does what we eat depend on where we live? Is food grown locally or imported to each country?
- How do the menus compare in nutritional value?
- Do customs about food vary in these different countries? If so, how?
- What do we mean by a poor diet or malnutrition?
- Why do some people eat more than they need? Does it matter?
- What can we do to help countries where people do not have enough to eat?

Suggestions for follow-up work
This introductory activity could lead on to project work, for example:
- Ask students to choose a particular country and find out how life for a family in that country differs from their own. What food is eaten? Who prepares it? When, where and how is it prepared and eaten? What foods are eaten for special celebrations?
- Get them to find out what organisations try to help countries where there is a food shortage, and how they help.
- Tell them that at least one child in three in poor countries is unhealthy because of poor nutrition. Ask them to write a story or poem to express their feelings about hunger.

- Invite students to make collections of pictures, cuttings and stories about food being used to celebrate festive/special occasions. Invite someone to describe a particular celebration/event they are familiar with.

SECTION 7: FOOD AND NUTRITION

Activity Sheet 58

Country cards

Photocopy and cut up before use

Countries

CHINA	**JAPAN**	**USA**
INDIA	**MOROCCO**	**UK**
	ITALY	

Menus

1 Tomato soup and bread
Lamb chops
Potatoes (boiled or mashed)
Peas and carrots
Apple crumble with custard/cream

2 Sweetcorn
Beefburgers and french fries
Side salad (mixed lettuce and tomato)
Chocolate fudge cake

3 Minestrone (mixed vegetable soup)
Pasta with tomato or meat sauce
Fruit

4 Cold meats
Rice or noodles with stir-fried and stewed vegetables (eg Chinese cabbage, spinach, aubergines, bean curd)
Lychees

5 Clear soup with chicken and mushrooms
Grilled fish
Boiled vegetables with chicken (carrots, potatoes, bamboo shoots)
Rice and pickled vegetables
Fruit

6 Salad of tomatoes, green peppers, onions and cucumber
Couscous (fine semolina/pasta) with lamb and vegetables
Bread
Fruit

7 Unleavened bread (baked or fried) or rice
Pickles and preserved vegetables and yoghurt
Stewed lentils
Cauliflower with spices
Okra with spices
Fruit

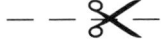

Answers

1 UK
2 USA
3 Italy
4 China
5 Japan
6 Morocco
7 India

SECTION 7: FOOD AND NUTRITION

ACTIVITY 59 — Food handling

Purpose
- To help students understand the main ways in which food can become contaminated
- To raise awareness of the need for food hygiene

Time needed 40 minutes

What you need Photographs and pictures of food handling (eg restaurants, shops, kitchens, cooks, butchers, supermarkets). Press cuttings – articles about outbreaks of food poisoning. A copy of Activity Sheet 59 for each student. Pens. Flipchart paper.

How you do it
1. Ask students to look at the pictures or photographs of food handlers. Can they suggest what food hygiene practices they have seen in these situations? Record their suggestions under the following headings: a) home, b) shops, c) restaurants.
2. Ask students why food hygiene is important. Point out that there are over 40,000 cases of food poisoning a year – many go unreported.
3. Divide the students into groups of three or four. Give each group a different selection of press cuttings about outbreaks of food poisoning and premises being closed down. Ask them to read these and discuss any experiences of food poisoning which they may have had. What were the main causes of infection and how might they have been prevented?
4. Ask each group to make a presentation of what they have learned (eg as a poster or chart).
5. Bring the class together to present their findings.
6. Give each student a copy of Activity Sheet 59 and compare the information on the sheet with their own findings.

Processing questions
- Were bacteria (germs) recognised as the main source of contamination of food?
- Are some bacteria useful in food production (eg making cheeses)?
- Why is it important to store food properly in a refrigerator?
- Why is it dangerous to reheat food?
- How can individuals help promote good food hygiene?
- What do we mean by 'shelf-life' of food?
- To whom can you complain or report poor food handling?

SECTION 7: FOOD AND NUTRITION

Suggestions for follow-up work

- Ask the students to collect information/leaflets about food handling for a display. Food Hygiene Guidelines (1990), produced by the Department of Health, lay down regulations for food handling in shops, market stalls and delivery vehicles. Advice on food handling is available from the Environmental Health Department of your local authority.
- Prepare and arrange for them to visit a supermarket to see food handling in action. Ask them to find out how much food is prepared and packaged at the shop, what the hygiene regulations are, and how often food is delivered.
- This workshop links with Activity 15 in the environment section.

Section 7: Food and Nutrition

Activity Sheet 59

Food handling

Food safety checklist

- Always wash your hands with hot soapy water before preparing food.
- Keep kitchens clean. Wash and dry utensils before each stage of preparing food.
- Keep pets out of kitchens.
- Cook food thoroughly.
- Do not reheat food more than once; if you do bacteria will multiply on the food.
- Keep fridge at the correct temperature (between 0 and 5 degrees C) to prevent bacteria multiplying. Freezers should be kept at −18 degrees C.
- Store raw and cooked foods on separate shelves in a fridge.
- Do not eat raw eggs.
- Check dates on goods; use within the recommended time.

SECTION 7: FOOD AND NUTRITION

ACTIVITY 60
Do you know what you're eating?

Purpose
- To encourage students to be critical of food labels
- To help students know what is in the food they eat

Time needed 30 minutes

What you need The labels or packaging from twenty different food products; list the ingredients from each label on cards, and put the names of the foods on separate cards. A copy of Activity Sheet 60 for each student.

How you do it

1 Divide the class into groups. Give each group four or five sets of ingredient cards and the corresponding food product cards. Ask them to try to match the product to the ingredient. Encourage groups to exchange their cards with those of other groups.

2 Ask students to choose one or two of the foods and to note:
What is the main ingredient?
Can they tell how much sugar or fat is in the product?
Have any nutrients been added?
What additives are used? Do they have E numbers?

3 Bring the class together to discuss labelling information, using Activity Sheet 60.

Processing questions
- Are there foods or ingredients they would like to find out more about?
- How *much* of any nutrient does a food contain?
- How easy is it to understand the labelling?
- Are additives useful? (Preservatives stop food spoiling and becoming unsafe to eat. Emulsifiers keep fat and water mixed.)
- Do people prefer highly coloured foods rather than natural-looking ones?
- What are E numbers? (E numbers mean that the EC have approved the use of the additive in food. Certain E numbers make food last longer. Some E numbers have been found to cause harm to certain people who are sensitive to them.)

Suggestions for follow-up work
- Ask students to interview someone who thinks organic food is a better choice. Get them to find out what s/he feels and why. Ask them to report the findings back to the class for comparison and discussion of the information they obtained.
- Compare the ingredients for a home-made cake (eg flour, eggs, sugar, milk, margarine, vanilla) with the ingredients in cake mixes. Do the same with other recipes for home-made foods and bought products.

Section 7: Food and Nutrition

ACTIVITY SHEET 60

Fact sheet

This kind of label would help you *know* what you are getting! How often do you look?

Carbohydrates include sugar we need to cut down and starch we need. Try to go for those which are mostly starch!

NUTRITION INFORMATION

100g (just under 4oz) gives you –

ENERGY	1440kJ/340kcals
PROTEIN	11.4g
CARBOHYDRATE	70.3g
of which sugars	6.1g
FAT	3.4g
of which saturates	0.5g
SODIUM	0.4g
FIBRE	12.7g

kJ = measure of energy

How many calories in 100g

This figure gives you an idea of how much salt is in the food. The higher the sodium, the more salt there is.

This 12.7g of fibre gives you nearly half of your target of 30g a day.

This figure tells you how much saturated fat is in 100g of the product. Go for the lowest amounts of this.

SECTION 7: FOOD AND NUTRITION

ACTIVITY 61 — *Junk food*

Purpose
- To help students distinguish between junk food and convenience food
- To help them recognise their own eating patterns
- To find ways of changing poor eating habits

Time needed 30 minutes

What you need A classroom display of pictures and advertisements for junk and convenience foods. A copy of Activity Sheets 61A and 61B for each student. Flipchart or board. Pens.

How you do it
1. Introduce the topic by inviting students to think how eating habits may have changed in Britain in recent years.
2. Brainstorm lists of foods students think of as junk and as convenience foods. Record their suggestions. At this stage make no comments.
3. Give each student a copy of Activity Sheet 61A to complete on their own.
4. Ask them to share their answers in groups of three or four.
5. Bring the class together to discuss their eating patterns to see how they relate to the list of junk/convenience foods from the brainstorm.

Processing questions
- How often do students eat snacks?
- Do they form the bulk of what they eat?
- Which are the foods they enjoy most?
- How much control over your diet do you have at home? Are there any ways you can get more control over what you eat?
- Is all convenience food junk? Give out Activity Sheet 61B if appropriate.
- Why do people use the fast-food chains such as Macdonalds and Pizza Hut? Are they good value?

Suggestions for follow-up work
- Ask students to collect ideas/recipes for healthy snacks. They could illustrate the suggestions with drawings or cuttings from magazines.
- Ask students to interview people from different generations to find out ways in which eating habits have changed in their lifetime. They should present their findings in the form of a newspaper report.

Section 7: Food and Nutrition

ACTIVITY SHEET 61A

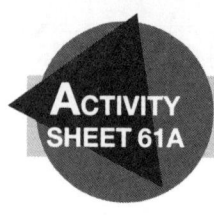

My eating profile

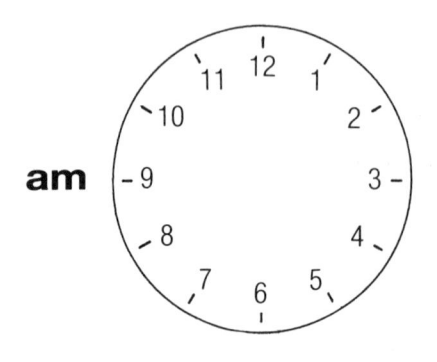

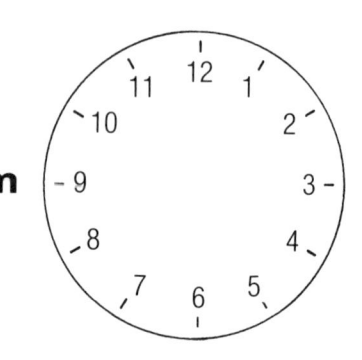

am (clock face)   **pm** (clock face)

Mark on the clocks the times when you had a snack or meal yesterday.

Fill in your answers to the following questions.

When did you eat? _ _ _ _ _ _ _ _ _ _ _ _ _

How often did you eat with other people? _ _ _ _ _ _ _ _ _ _

How often did you eat alone? _ _ _ _ _ _ _ _ _ _ _ _

Did you eat between main meals? _ _ _ _ _ _ _ _ _ _ _

If 'Yes', what did you have? _ _ _ _ _ _ _ _ _ _ _ _

Were you hungry each time you ate? _ _ _ _ _ _ _ _ _ _

Were you doing something else when you ate (eg watching TV, doing homework, meeting friends)? _ _ _ _ _ _ _ _

Were you in a rush when you ate? _ _ _ _ _ _ _ _ _ _ _

Do you prefer long-lasting snacks or several quick snacks during a day? _ _ _ _ _ _ _ _ _ _

Do you buy your own snacks or are they bought or prepared for you? _ _ _ _ _

Look at the answers you have given above. Are there any eating habits which you would like to change? _ _ _ _ _ _ _ _

If your answer is 'Yes', what is it you want to change and why? _ _ _ _ _ _

© A Picture of Health   Permission to photocopy this page for participant use

Section 7: Food and Nutrition

Activity Sheet 61B

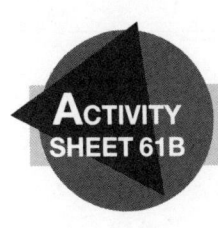

Fact sheet

HEALTHY CONVENIENCE FOODS

Fresh
All fruit and vegetables
Skimmed or semi-skimmed milk
Low-fat, unsweetened yogurt
Wholemeal bread

Frozen
All frozen vegetables (no batter or sauces)
Fish (no batter or sauces)

Tinned
Sardines
Tuna
Tomatoes
Green beans
Sweetcorn
Carrots
Baked beans

Dried
Dried fruit
Nuts (unsalted)
Wholemeal pasta
Brown rice
Dried beans

CAN YOU THINK OF OTHERS?

Foods to avoid
Chips
Burgers
Sausages

SECTION 7: FOOD AND NUTRITION

ACTIVITY 62
What's right for me?

Purpose
- To help students decide whether to make changes in their eating habits
- To make them aware of the three basic body types
- To help them realise that proper balance between food intake and energy output will result in weight control
- To help them understand the ineffectiveness of crash diets
- To share ideas about effective weight control

Time needed 40 minutes

What you need A copy of Activity Sheets 62A and 62B for each student. Pens.

How you do it It is important that teachers are sensitive to any obese students in their class and amend the exercises accordingly.

1. Ask students to look at the pictures of the young people on Activity Sheet 62A and complete it for themselves.
2. Ask how they can decide what is the correct weight for them. They can just look in the mirror! However, people tend to be over-critical and feel they don't measure up to the images given in films and magazines. They can look at *height/weight charts*, which give average weights based on height, age, sex. Or they can take the *skinfold measurements* at the back of the right arm, in front of the arm, on the back, thigh and abdomen (the pinch test).
3. Hand out Fact Sheet 62B. Ask them to read through this, making sure they understand what is meant by the different body types and the metabolic rate.
4. Encourage discussion.

Processing questions
- Can students decide which body type they are? Are they a combination? If so, which?
- Can they think of someone who eats and eats and stays the same weight? Why is this?
- What are the reasons for the increasing number of overweight people in our society today?
- Is too much emphasis placed on being slim?
- Are there dangers in crash diets which offer huge weight losses in a short time? How can you evaluate them?
- Are some diets harmful for growing people?
- Can it help to have a support group if they want to lose weight?
- What are the ways in which people can increase body weight if they feel they lack muscle?
- How easy is it to change eating patterns? Brainstorm ideas for sensible dieting.

Section 7: Food and Nutrition

Suggestions for follow-up work
- If they decide they want to change their eating pattern, suggest that they follow the action plan, in Activity Sheet 70.
- Divide the class into two groups:
  Group 1 – Students design a one-day meal plan for a 14-year-old girl trying to maintain her weight.
  Group 2 – Students design a one-day meal plan for a 14-year-old boy trying to gain weight.
  Display the suggestions.

SECTION 7: FOOD AND NUTRITION

ACTIVITY SHEET 62A

Pictures

Do you ever feel like the people in these pictures?

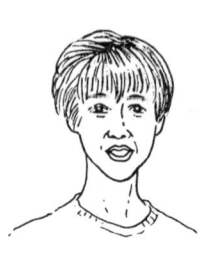

I wish I could put on weight. I feel such a wimp.

I find it hard to eat sensibly. All my friends go for the french fries and fizzy drinks.

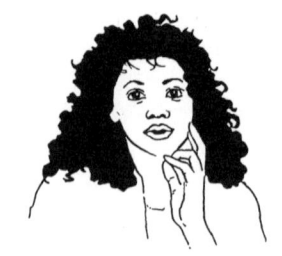

Whenever I feel miserable, I just sit and eat!

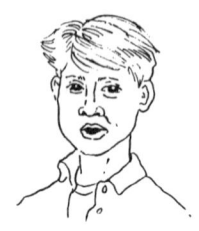

I want to look attractive.

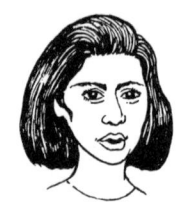

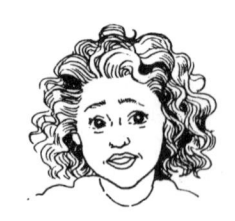

I worry because I know I am overweight – and all my family are fat!

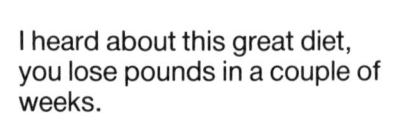

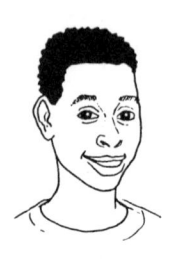

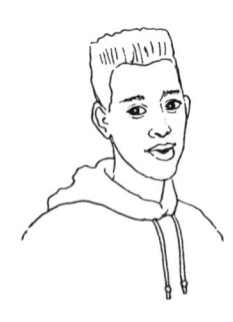

I heard about this great diet, you lose pounds in a couple of weeks.

I have already got a mouth full of fillings!

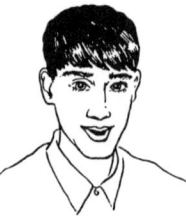

I want to cut down on fats and be a vegetarian.

182 © A Picture of Health   Permission to photocopy this page for participant use

Section 7: Food and Nutrition

Fill in what you would say about your eating pattern

....
....
....
....
....
....
....
....

Ask yourself the following questions before you make any decision to change your weight

Do I feel OK about my weight?

How can I tell if I'm the correct weight?

Would I be more active if I lost weight?

Would I like to put on more weight?

Would I feel less self-conscious if I lost or gained weight?

Are there things I cannot do because of my weight?

SECTION 7: FOOD AND NUTRITION

ACTIVITY SHEET 62B

Fact sheet

Pinch test – how to measure your body fat

Nearly half our body fat is found just under the surface of the skin. Measuring the amount of fat in certain places is a good way to determine your overall body fat. This is done by getting someone to pinch the back of your right arm *gently* and with a ruler measure the width of the pinched skin. You could do the same with the back, the abdomen and the inner thigh. Readings of over 2.5cm for a girl and 2cm for a boy mean the amount of fat is high.

What are body types?

Ectomorph
These people are thin and slender. They have a light body build with very little fat.

Mesomorph
These people have a medium body frame, often quite muscular.

Endomorph
These people are heavy, rounded in build.

Most of us are a combination of these or are more one type than another. It is helpful to recognise your body build before you decide to slim. An endomorph will never end up an ectomorph!

Why can some people eat and eat and still be thin?

This depends on your METABOLIC RATE. This is the speed at which we burn up the energy we take in as food. Your body needs energy to maintain its vital functions – blood circulation, digestion, respiration and maintaining temperature. Even when you are asleep you are using up some energy. People with a high rate burn off energy rapidly and stay thin. Those with a slow rate use up energy slowly and need to take more exercise.

How much energy do we need to stay healthy?

The daily energy requirement for a 13–15-year-old boy is 12,000 kJ, for a girl the same age it is 9,200 kJ. The energy in food is measured in kiloJoules or calories and the energy your body uses up is measured in kiloJoules.

WEIGHT STAYS SAME
Energy from food and drink = Energy used in activities in daily life

WEIGHT GOES DOWN
Less food + More activity

WEIGHT GOES UP
More food + Less activity

You can't control your weight by diet alone. Try to find activities you *enjoy* which use up energy. Find out how much energy different activities use up.

SECTION 7: FOOD AND NUTRITION

ACTIVITY 63 — *I can't refuse*

Purpose
- To help students see how negative self-talk affects behaviour
- To offer students strategies for changing to positive self-talk

Time needed 30 minutes

What you need A copy of Activity Sheets 63A and 63B for each student

How you do it
1. Hand out Activity Sheet 63A. Ask students to imagine they are in the situations described on it. All the situations are to do with food. They have to make a quick decision. In pairs, ask them to share with each other what they would do and why they would decide to act in this way.
2. In the whole class, share the answers and the strategies students used to cope with the situation.

Processing questions
- Did people come up with similar answers?
- How easy is it to act in our own best interests when that may offend others?
- Do we have a right to say 'No' without feeling guilty? Have they been in situations like this?
- What were the consequences of their decisions likely to be?
- Were students able to be assertive in the way they responded?

How you do it continued
3. Ask students to look at the situations again and think about the kind of things that might run through their heads as they responded to them. Introduce the concept of 'self-talk' and the way this can be negative or positive. Was it negative self-talk that prevented them from responding assertively in any of the situations? Share examples.
4. How can they change negative self-talk into positive? Ask students to look at the statements of young people on Activity Sheet 63B and to turn them into positive self-talk.
5. Bring the class together to discuss ways of challenging unhelpful self-talk: remember your right to be assertive, replace negative thoughts with positive, avoid labelling yourself, stop foreseeing disaster, stop the thought.

Suggestions for follow-up work This activity links with activities on assertiveness in Section 1 and gives students the opportunity to practise using role play situations.

Section 7: Food and Nutrition

ACTIVITY SHEET 63A

I can't refuse

Imagine you are in the situations below.

What would you do?

Why would you decide in this way?

1. The parents of your friend have invited you to dinner at their house. They offer you fried chicken, baked potatoes with sour cream and butter, and vegetables covered in a creamy sauce. The pudding is a chocolate gateau. You are trying to lose weight.

2. You are out with a group of friends. You are trying hard to develop a healthy pattern of eating. All your friends are eating chips and burgers.

3. You go to visit an elderly relative. S/he looks forward to your visit and has put on a special tea for you with lots of home-made cakes. You are conscious about your weight and want to eat sensibly.

Share your answers with your partner. What would be the consequences of your decisions? What might you feel?

SECTION 7: FOOD AND NUTRITION

Challenging negative self-talk

ACTIVITY SHEET 63B

SITUATION	You are offered a doughnut smothered in sugar
RESPONSE thought/self-talk	I can't refuse when they bought it for me
CONSEQUENCE	You eat it and feel angry with yourself

What you think can decide what you feel and do. What we tell ourselves or how we label ourselves can have an effect on how we behave.

Look at the young people in the pictures and notice what they are saying to themselves. Can you change their negative self-talk to positive? How have they labelled themselves?

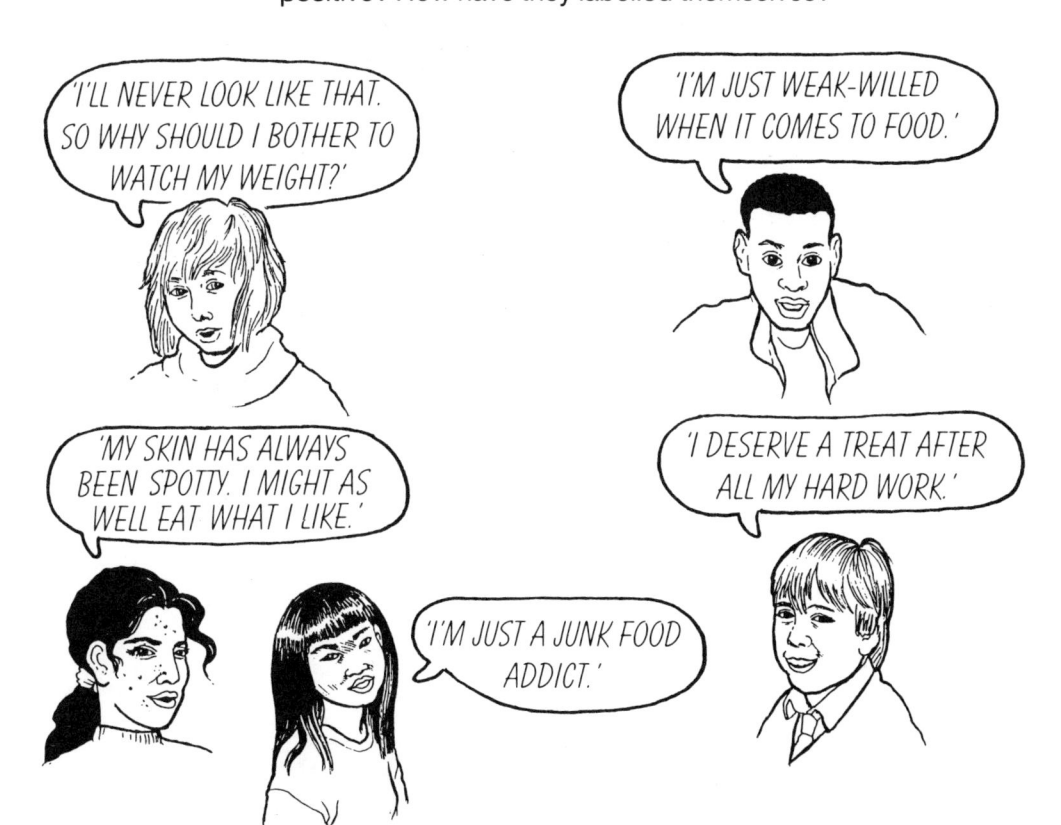

'I'LL NEVER LOOK LIKE THAT. SO WHY SHOULD I BOTHER TO WATCH MY WEIGHT?'

'I'M JUST WEAK-WILLED WHEN IT COMES TO FOOD.'

'MY SKIN HAS ALWAYS BEEN SPOTTY. I MIGHT AS WELL EAT WHAT I LIKE.'

'I DESERVE A TREAT AFTER ALL MY HARD WORK.'

'I'M JUST A JUNK FOOD ADDICT.'

© A Picture of Health   Permission to photocopy this page for participant use

SECTION 7: FOOD AND NUTRITION

ACTIVITY 64 — *A school survey*

Purpose
- To enable students to find out more about the school meals service in their school
- To develop skills of investigation and enquiry

Time needed Variable

What you need A copy of Activity Sheet 64 for each student. Flipchart or board.

How you do it
1. Explain to students that this activity will give them an opportunity to find out more about the school meals service in their canteen.
2. Brainstorm the kind of information they would like to have.
3. Ask them who will need to be interviewed to get the information. Record the ideas. Divide the class into small groups. Each is to take responsibility for a specific aspect of the enquiry.
4. Give out Activity Sheet 64. Each group is to work through the sheet, preparing their questions.
5. Bring the suggestions together and arrange how students will collect the information. Decide when they will report back on their findings and how this will be done.

Processing questions
- Is any special permission needed before carrying out a survey?
- How will they check whether people are willing to be interviewed?
- How are answers to be recorded?
- Is everyone to be involved?
- Who else can help with the survey?

Suggestions for follow-up work
- Review the learning from the survey. What have the students learnt about the school meals service?
- Discuss what has been learnt about carrying out surveys. Do students think there are further investigations to carry out?
- This activity could be developed using the visitor technique outlined in Activity 39 of the family life education section, with the class inviting the school meals supervisor as the visitor.

SECTION 7: FOOD AND NUTRITION

ACTIVITY SHEET 64

An interview checksheet

STEP BY STEP GUIDE

STEP 1 What do you want to find out? Write down as many things as possible.

STEP 2 Who do you need to interview to get the information?

STEP 3 Decide on the most important aspects to ask each person and turn these into questions.

STEP 4 Check the wording of the questions. Can they be easily understood? Can they be answered with a simple 'Yes' or 'No'? You will find out more if you ask questions beginning with 'When', 'Who', 'Which', 'Why' and 'Where'.

STEP 5 Have you thought about the order of the questions? Does each naturally follow another?

STEP 6 'Pilot' or try these out with one or two people to make sure you get the kind of information you are looking for.

STEP 7 Decide who is going to ask the questions, where you are going to ask them and how you are going to record the answers.

SECTION 8

Health-related exercise

SECTION 8: HEALTH-RELATED EXERCISE

ACTIVITY 65 — Why exercise?

Purpose	• To discuss the reasons for exercising and keeping fit
Time needed	20 minutes
What you need	A copy of Activity Sheet 65 for each participant. Pens.
How you do it	1 Point out that people take varying amounts of exercise. Some seem really to enjoy it. Others have got it into their heads that exercise is not for them. 2 Give students Activity Sheet 65, and ask them to complete it on their own. 3 Form the class into groups of four to share their results.
Processing questions	• What were the most popular reasons given for/against exercising? • Did they disagree with any statement? Are they all true? • Do people choose different activities for different reasons? • Do they know the effects of different types of exercises – for example, which activities build strong muscles?
Suggestions for follow-up work	In this section, Activity 66 gives more information about the benefits of exercising. Activity 71 encourages students to overcome the barriers against keeping fit.

Section 8: Health-Related Exercise

Activity Sheet 65

Why exercise?

The following comments about the reasons for exercising or keeping fit were all made by young people. Some also point out why they don't exercise.

If you were deciding whether to exercise or not, which three comments would be *most important* to you? Mark these with a tick. Which three would be *least important*? Mark these with a cross.

Can you think of any other reasons for or against exercising?

'Exercise makes your heart work harder.'

'The money puts me off. You feel daft without the right gear.'

'Everyone seems to be going to aerobics and keep-fit classes. I think they're doing it to be thin and attractive rather than healthy.'

'If you're shy and you go out to meet people doing sport, then you're getting fit and you're coming out of yourself more.'

'If you can run round a field you feel you've achieved something.'

'Exercise is good for you if you're dieting or trying to keep your weight constant.'

'People play sport because they enjoy it.'

'Exercise works your muscles, makes you stronger.'

'I went along and did it just one lesson and I was absolutely useless at it. I wasn't keen to do it any more.'

'Having a game of football or tennis is a social thing as well.'

'It's good to do something completely different from what you do the rest of the day.'

'Exercise takes all the tension out of you. You feel more relaxed after it.'

'If you do exercises, it gives you more energy.'

'When you've put on weight, you feel frumpy. You think "I'm not going swimming because everybody's going to laugh at me, 'cause I'm fat."'

'Young men join in weight-lifting just for their appearance.'

'If you're fit, you're more likely to be mentally fit as well.'

Another reason for exercising is ....

....

Another reason for not exercising is ....

....

SECTION 8: HEALTH-RELATED EXERCISE

ACTIVITY 66
There's more than one way

Purpose	• To identify the range of exercises/sports available • To discuss the appropriateness of these for different people • To help students understand the three 'S' factors: suppleness, stamina and strength
Time needed	30 minutes
What you need	Large sheets of flipchart paper. Gummed stars or shapes in three different colours. Activity Sheet 66. Felt-tip pens.
How you do it	1 Divide the class into groups of four or five and give each a sheet of flipchart paper. Ask half the groups to brainstorm all the sports that girls can play (both in and away from school) and the other half to brainstorm all the sports that boys can play. 2 Give each group a copy of Activity Sheet 66. Talk through the three 'S' factors. Give each group several gummed stars or shapes: one colour for Stamina, one for Suppleness and one for Strength. Ask them to decide for each activity which of the three 'S' factors it would help to build, and to stick the appropriate coloured star or stars next to each. 3 After 10 minutes, compare the lists. As the groups report back, list each of the sports and mark B next to it if it is mentioned as a sport boys can play, and G if mentioned as a sport girls can play. Put a mark (eg with coloured pens or chalk) next to each sport to show whether they think it builds stamina, strength or suppleness.
Processing questions	• How many sports are considered appropriate to both boys and girls? Has this changed in any way over the past ten years? • Are there some sports that girls cannot play? Why? • Which sports tend to appeal to girls and which to boys? • Do the sports chosen by boys or girls tend to build up certain 'S' factors rather than others?
Suggestions for follow-up work	Ask each student to interview three people of different ages about the types of activities they do to keep fit. Possible questions are: How much time per week do they spend on them? Did they use to be more physically active? What do they like or dislike about exercising?

SECTION 8: HEALTH-RELATED EXERCISE

ACTIVITY SHEET 66

Fitness is having stamina, suppleness and strength

Stamina

This is what you need to be able to keep going, when running or walking briskly, without getting tired and puffed very quickly. Stamina is useful when you're in a hurry to get somewhere or you have to carry out a vigorous activity for a long period of time. The best activities for improving stamina are fairly energetic, make you slightly out of breath and keep you moving for 20 minutes or more. This type of exercise is often called 'aerobic' exercise because you breathe in enough oxygen to supply your working muscles. The lungs and heart work hard to supply the extra oxygen needed.

Examples of exercises: jogging, swimming, brisk walking, aerobics, cycling

Suppleness

When you have this, you are able to bend, stretch, twist and turn through a full range of movement. If you're supple, you're less likely to get injured or to have sore muscles or lower back pain. People with good flexibility can move gracefully.

Examples of exercises: gymnastics, yoga, dancing, judo

Strength

Having strength enables you to exert force – for pushing, pulling and lifting. You need strength all the time, even to move around and carry books! Muscular strength helps to reduce tiredness and develop good posture. It can also help to prevent muscle injuries, soreness and back pain.

Examples of exercises: rowing, digging the garden, weight-lifting

Section 8: Health-Related Exercise

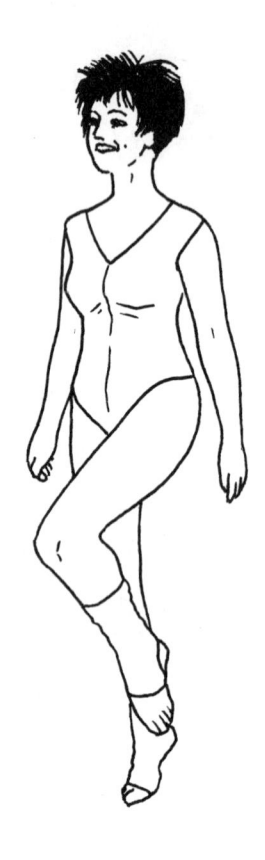

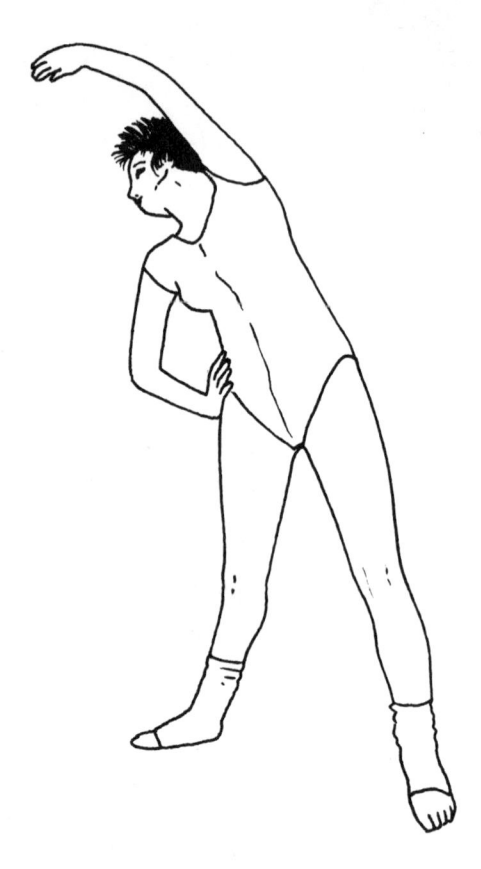

Here are some benefits you can get from being fit

nervous system reacts more quickly, and co-ordination and reaction time improves

lungs work more efficiently and have greater capacity

muscles strengthen and tone

bones and joints strengthen

body becomes firm and trim

person feels more alert and can concentrate better

better blood circulation improves complexion

heart works more efficiently

posture improves

body becomes more flexible

Anyone can be physically fit – regardless of age or physical ability. People who have never been physically active before are getting into exercise programmes and sports, and are amazed at what they can do. People with disabilities, whether mental or physical, are becoming involved in recreational and competitive sports programmes, such as swimming, basketball, table tennis and marathons.

SECTION 8: HEALTH-RELATED EXERCISE

ACTIVITY 67 — *What is there to do?*

Purpose
- To encourage students to investigate the sports facilities that are provided in their community

Time needed 20 minutes plus time outside the session to carry out the project

What you need General information about the sports facilities provided by the local council – from the library, local council offices or Citizens' Advice Bureau. Local newspapers and Yellow Pages.

How you do it
1. Hand out information about sports facilities which are available locally.
2. Divide the class into pairs. Ask students to choose one of the sports facilities for a detailed study. It should be a place which they can visit after school.
3. Get the group as a whole to list all the basic information which they need to find out, for example opening times, entrance charges, details of activities and facilities provided and any special features.
4. Ask each pair to list questions they might ask about the service provided, such as:
   ○ Is it easy to get to by public transport?
   ○ Do the entrance charges seem high or about right?
   ○ Do the facilities seem well used? By whom?
   ○ Does it make special provision for the unemployed, students, senior citizens, the handicapped, young children?
   ○ Is it well decorated and in good repair?
5. Ask them to visit the facility before the next session and if possible to interview a number of people there, asking how often they use the facility, whether they have travelled a long way to get there, how satisfied they are with the place and the service offered.
6. Each pair then presents a report to the group.

Processing questions
- Did they find it easy to get information?
- Would they do anything differently another time?
- Are there any sports facilities which seem to be lacking in our community?
- Are there any particular groups of people who are missing out?
- What improvements would they recommend?

Suggestions for follow-up work They could make the information available to others, for example by designing a display in the school or writing a letter to the head of the local leisure and recreation department with specific requests or suggestions (address will be listed in the telephone book under the name of the local authority).

Section 8: Health-Related Exercise

Activity 68: Taking your pulse rate

Purpose
- To teach students how to monitor their pulse rate

Time needed 5–10 minutes

What you need Watches or a clock with a second hand

How you do it

1. Explain that in order to make sure that the aerobic exercises they do are effective and safe, they need to be able to check their 'resting' and 'working' pulse rates. Ask if anyone knows how. If so, encourage her/him to explain how to the group. Otherwise take them through the following process.

2. The resting pulse should be taken when they are sitting down and relaxed.

3. Ask them to find their pulse with their fingers (not thumbs as the thumb has its own pulse and this will confuse them). There are various places on the body where the heartbeat can be counted. The easiest to find are on the inside of either wrist or at the side of the neck (in the corner under the jaw on either side). Demonstrate where on yourself. Check that everyone can find their pulse.

4. Using a watch or clock with a second hand, wait until the second hand reaches a point from which it is easy to calculate 15 seconds (ie the 3, 6, 9 or 12 o'clock position).

5. Ask each student to start counting their heartbeats for 15 seconds. Multiply that number by 4 to work out their resting pulse rate. The fitter the person is, the lower it will be. Generally a person with a resting pulse rate below 60 beats per minute has a healthy cardio-respiratory system. A very fit athlete may have a resting rate of 40 beats to the minute.

Processing questions
- Why is it useful to be able to monitor your pulse rate?

Suggestions for follow-up work
- Encourage them to take their pulse before and immediately after some form of aerobic exercising. See Activity Sheet 69B.
- Plan a fitness programme for themselves over a month (see Activity 70). Get them to keep an exercise diary (Activity Sheet 69A). Get them to note their resting pulse rate at the beginning and end of the programme.

SECTION 8: HEALTH-RELATED EXERCISE

ACTIVITY 69 — How fit are you?

Purpose	• To increase students' awareness of their level of fitness • To motivate students to exercise in their own time
Time needed	10 minutes initially, then 5 minutes daily by each person. At a session the following week, 15 minutes.
What you need	A copy of Activity Sheets 69A and 69B for each student

How you do it	1 Give each student a copy of Activity Sheets 69A and 69B.
	2 Explain that Activity Sheet 69A is an exercise diary. Ask them to fill it in each day for a week. At the end of each day, they should fill in the types of activity undertaken, how long they spent on each and any comments about how they felt as a result. Remind them to include activities such as walking to school or cycling on a paper round as well as more formal sports sessions.
	3 Also ask them to try out at home the fitness tests on Activity Sheet 69B.
	4 At a session the following week, write the following questions on the board. Ask them to find a partner and interview each other, using the questions as a guideline:
	   ○ What did they learn from keeping the diary (eg were they surprised at the amount of exercise they did)?
	   ○ What time of day did they tend to exercise?
	   ○ What did they enjoy most?
	   ○ Which type of exercises did they do most – ones that build strength, stamina or suppleness?
	   ○ Which type of exercises do they need more of?
	   ○ What were their reasons for not exercising?
	   ○ Did keeping a diary influence what they did?
	   ○ What were the results of doing the fitness tests?
	5 In the whole group, encourage a general discussion on the process of keeping a diary and testing oneself. Try to avoid putting anyone on the spot.

Processing questions	• Did they find in their pairs that they had anything in common? If so, would they be willing to talk about it? • What are the possible benefits and drawbacks of keeping a diary? • Have they learnt anything which others might find useful?
Suggestions for follow-up work	Activity 70 could be a useful next step, helping them to set their own targets for improvement.

SECTION 8: HEALTH-RELATED EXERCISE

ACTIVITY SHEET 69A

An exercise diary

		Activities	Time taken	Comments
Examples		10 mins	Cycling	Did 2 miles. Felt puffed going up Wellard Hill.
MONDAY	am			
	pm			
	evening			
TUESDAY	am			
	pm			
	evening			
WEDNESDAY	am			
	pm			
	evening			
THURSDAY	am			
	pm			
	evening			
FRIDAY	am			
	pm			
	evening			
SATURDAY	am			
	pm			
	evening			
SUNDAY	am			
	pm			
	evening			

© A Picture of Health   Permission to photocopy this page for participant use

Section 8: Health-Related Exercise

How fit are you?

Try out these tests to check your fitness.

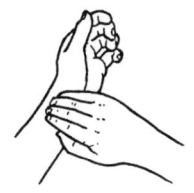

STAMINA

Check how quickly your pulse rate returns to normal after exercising hard. The quicker it recovers, the fitter you are. Check it *immediately* after exercising, keeping walking on the spot, as the pulse rate slows down very quickly when you stop an exercise.

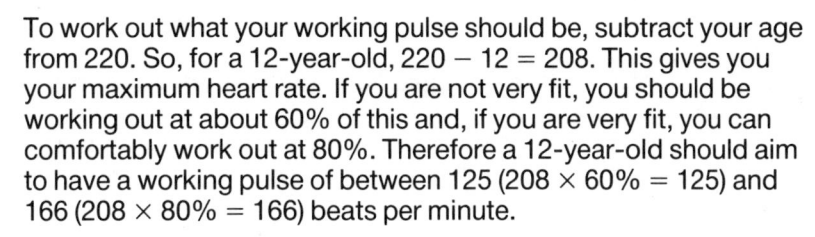

To work out what your working pulse should be, subtract your age from 220. So, for a 12-year-old, 220 − 12 = 208. This gives you your maximum heart rate. If you are not very fit, you should be working out at about 60% of this and, if you are very fit, you can comfortably work out at 80%. Therefore a 12-year-old should aim to have a working pulse of between 125 (208 × 60% = 125) and 166 (208 × 80% = 166) beats per minute.

Can you work out the target pulse rates (between 60% and 80%) for a 13-year-old? (The answer is at the bottom of this activity sheet.)

The Step Test

1. Place your right foot on the first step
2. Place your left foot on the second step
3. Take your right foot to the second step, so feet are together
4. Step down with left foot to the first step
5. Step down with right foot to the ground
6. Take your left foot down so feet are together

Repeat the stepping sequence to music for 3 minutes. Take your pulse before you start and immediately after you stop.

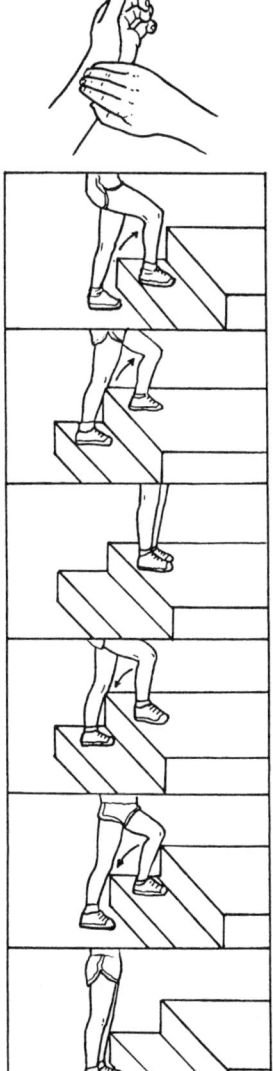

SECTION 8: HEALTH-RELATED EXERCISE

SUPPLENESS

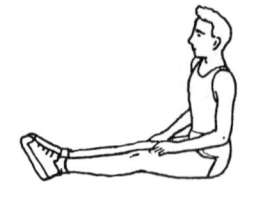

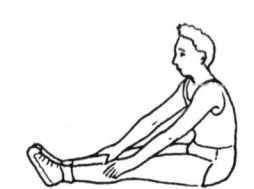

Sit on the floor with your legs straight out in front of you. Place your hands on top of your thighs and slowly and smoothly slide your hands down your legs as far as you can comfortably reach. Hold it for a count of 20. Don't force yourself. You are very flexible if you can hook your hands over your toes, and not bad if you can reach your ankles.

STRENGTH

You can test the strength of your arms by doing push-ups.

1. Place hands under your shoulders, legs straight together and toes to the ground
2. Push with your arms until they are straight
3. Then lower your body, keeping the back in a straight line, until your elbows are at 90 degrees and your arms are parallel to the ground
4. Repeat push-ups rhythmically and continuously

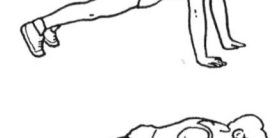

If you are 13, an average score is 4 for girls and 11 for boys. An excellent score would be 21 for girls and 39 for boys. Something to aim for?

Try partial curl-ups to test the strength of your abdominal muscles. These are done rhythmically at a rate of about 20 per minute.

1. Lie on your back, knees bent, heels on the ground and feet 3 to 5 inches apart. Press the small of your back into the floor.
2. Put your hands on the top of your thighs. Lifting just your head and shoulders off the floor, slide your fingers along your thighs as far as is comfortable.
3. Then uncurl slowly back to the lying position.

An average score for 13-year-olds is 28 for boys and 22 for girls. An excellent score for both would be 50.

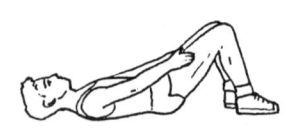

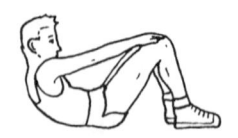

Target pulse rates question

The target pulse rates for a 13-year-old would be between 124 and 166 beats per minute.

$$220 - 13 = 207 \times 60\% = 124$$
$$\times 80\% = 166$$

Section 8: Health-Related Exercise

Activity 70: Choosing what's right for you

Purpose
- To encourage students to begin to determine their own priorities in keeping fit
- To help them decide on an action plan related to keeping fit
- To help them practise listening and clarifying skills

Time needed 30 minutes, plus 15 minutes at a later session

What you need A copy of Activity Sheet 70 for each student. Pens.

How you do it
1. Give each student a copy of Activity Sheet 70 and allow her/him 5 minutes to complete the 'shopping' task at the top of the page.
2. Get them, in pairs, to discuss questions a, b and c on the sheet.
3. Ask each person to think about something which s/he is going to do before the next session concerning her/his own fitness. It might be to follow an exercise programme on a video at home, to visit a local leisure centre to find out what amenities are available, to play a certain sport at school or to go for a cycle ride.
4. Ask them to complete the action plan on the activity sheet.
5. Explain that it often helps us to carry something out if we make a contract to do it. Ask them to choose a partner and to talk through what they have written. Allow 5 minutes each.
6. Get them to help one another in turn to be clear about what they are going to do. Each should listen for any signs of doubt, such as 'perhaps' and 'if I feel like it', and check out with one another whether they are unsure. Try to help them to be as specific as possible: not 'I'm going to cycle more', but 'Saturday I'll cycle to my friend's house rather than asking for a lift.'
7. Decide on a time (possibly in the same session the following week) when the pair will get together again to see how they have each got on.

Processing questions
- How easy was it to identify something they were going to do?
- Would anyone be willing to say what they plan to do?

  (At the next session)
- What has anyone learnt from this?
- What would they do differently another time?

Suggestions for follow-up work Repeat the process, so that students get used to the idea of trying again and developing further.

Section 8: Health-Related Exercise

ACTIVITY SHEET 70

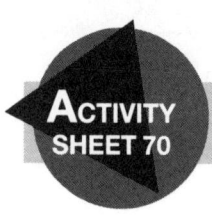

Choosing what's right for you

You are in a futuristic shop where you can buy almost anything to help you improve your physical fitness. Everything for sale in this shop comes in three sizes: large at £10, medium at £5 and small at £2. You have £50 to spend. Decide which items and at what size you would buy.

ITEMS

- activities to lose weight
- activities to relieve tension
- activities to develop strong muscles
- activities to give more energy
- time to do more physical activity
- motivation to get started on an exercise programme
- will-power to keep to a regular exercise programme
- facilities for exercising
- friends to do activities with

Talk with someone else about the following questions:

1. What items did you purchase and why?
2. How might the items improve your level of fitness?
3. What are the benefits you could get?

Section 8: Health-Related Exercise

ACTION PLAN

I AM GOING TO ....

....

WHEN? ....

....

HOW? ....

....

WHAT HELP WILL I NEED? ....

....

HOW WILL I KNOW I'VE BEEN SUCCESSFUL? ....

....

....

HOW AM I LIKELY TO STOP MYSELF FROM
SUCCEEDING? ....

....

....

WHAT WILL BE THE BENEFITS OF SUCCEEDING? ....

....

....

HOW SHALL I GIVE MYSELF A REWARD? ....

....

....

SECTION 8: HEALTH-RELATED EXERCISE

ACTIVITY SHEET 71

What's stopping you?

Purpose	• To discuss what stops people from exercising • To identify strategies to overcome this
Time needed	30 minutes
What you need	Activity Sheet 71, photocopied on to card, and cut up. You need enough for each student to have either an EXCUSE or an ANSWER. Index cards. Pens.
How you do it	1 Give out one card to each student. 2 Explain that half the students have a card that outlines an excuse that someone may give for not exercising, and the other half a card giving a possible answer to the excuse. 3 Students move around the room trying to find the person who has the card which matches theirs. They do this by each reading what is on their card and seeing if the answer corresponds. 4 Once everyone has a partner, ask them to sit down and discuss what is on their cards. Is the excuse often used? Would people take any notice of the reply? 5 Ask each pair to think up a short case-study about someone who uses the excuse on their card, for example: 'Sharon is 13. She makes every excuse she can to get out of PE. She always says to her friends that she's not the sporty type.' 6 Ask them to write their case-study on an index card and exchange this with another pair. 7 Students then discuss the case-study they have been given, deciding: ○ What could the person her/himself do to overcome her/his 'block'/ and keep fit? ○ What could her/his friends or other people do to help? ○ What social changes might help – for example facilities or images in the media? 8 Get each pair to join another to form groups of four to discuss the strategies they identified. How do these compare with the answer given on the original card? Ask for feedback in the whole group.
Processing questions	• Which excuses are the most difficult to overcome? • At some time or another, do we all make excuses for not taking exercise? • What helps to overcome this?
Suggestions for follow-up work	Ask students to design a poster that encourages others to take exercise.

SECTION 8: HEALTH-RELATED EXERCISE

ACTIVITY 71 — *What's stopping you?*

Excuse   'It's too much like hard work. I'd never keep it up.'

Answer   It won't seem like hard work if you choose an exercise you enjoy and build up gradually. As you get better you'll enjoy it even more and you won't want to give it up.

Excuse   'What I need is relaxation.'

Answer   Exercise can be just the thing to help you relax. It takes your mind off any problems you might have. You'll notice the relaxing effects of some kinds of exercise even while you're doing them. And afterwards, you'll feel warm, comfortable and relaxed. Exercising can lift depression. You'll probably find it helps you sleep better too.

Excuse   'I haven't got time. I'm too busy.'

Answer   Just 20 minutes, two or three times a week, can keep you fit. It will also help you to feel less restless and better able to concentrate on schoolwork or other demanding mental tasks.

Excuse   'But doesn't it have to hurt to do you any good?'

Answer   No. If it hurts then you're pushing yourself too hard. If you're uncomfortably out of breath, then slow down. If you're in pain, stop. When you're exercising you should be aware of how your body feels and not push it too far.

Excuse   'I'm too fat for that kind of thing.'

Answer   Exercising helps you get slim and stay slim by burning off more calories. If you use up more energy through exercise than you eat in food, your body will start using up its own energy stores and fat will start to disappear.

© A Picture of Health   Permission to photocopy this page for participant use

SECTION 8: HEALTH-RELATED EXERCISE

Excuse 'I'd be too embarrassed.'

Answer Don't let embarrassment put you off exercise. Focus on your activity and don't think about how you look or perform. People of all shapes and sizes enjoy exercising. Choose an activity that's right for you. When you're fit, you will feel good about yourself and find it easier to approach people or take on difficult tasks.

Excuse 'I'm not a sporty person.'

Answer Maybe you've just not found a sport that's right for you. There are so many different activities, you're sure to be able to find one you enjoy. If you like dancing and music, think about aerobics. If you like competition, join a sports league. If you like to be on your own, try cycling or brisk walking. You'll soon find out how it feels to be able to say 'I'm a very active person!'

Excuse 'I keep meaning to start, but somehow never get round to it.'

Answer All you have to do is set a date, time and place and get started. Think positively. Imagine a fit you – relaxed, energetic, attractive, self-confident. What are you waiting for?

Excuse 'I couldn't do it on my own.'

Answer You don't have to. Taking part in a sport or exercising with others will give you an opportunity to meet people and make new friends. Or you could persuade people who are already your friends to exercise with you. Try to involve them.

Excuse 'If I can't do it properly, then what's the point of doing it at all?'

Answer You don't have to go into serious training or get super-fit to gain from exercising. Regular activity for just 20 or 30 minutes, two or three times a week, will go a long way towards helping you stay in good shape.

Excuse 'I couldn't bear all the injuries.'

Answer There don't have to be any. Don't push yourself too hard. Listen to what your body is telling you. Exercise builds strong muscles which protect you from injury.

SECTION 8: HEALTH-RELATED EXERCISE

ACTIVITY SHEET 72
A stressful wordsearch

Purpose
- To help students recognise the different signs of stress
- To discuss ways of preventing stress

Time needed 30–40 minutes

What you need A copy of Activity Sheet 72 for each student. Cut off the answer before distributing them. Pens.

How you do it

1. Ask students to form pairs. Ask each pair to think of a time when they have felt stressed. Explain that this might be because they had something to do which they felt was very demanding, or they may not have had enough to do – that can be stressful. It may have only lasted a short while. It may have gone on for several weeks or months. How did they feel? What 'symptoms' were there? How did they tend to behave? Ask them to jot down their answers.

2. Give each pair a copy of Activity Sheet 72, explaining that it contains twenty-eight words and terms which can be signs or symptoms of stress. Can they find them? Hand out the answer when they have finished or if they seem to be getting stuck.

3. How did these words compare with the ones they had written down that were based on their own experiences? Ask them to underline any words on Activity Sheet 72 which they had mentioned in their own discussions.

Processing questions
- Were they confused by any of the words or terms on Activity Sheet 72? Were they unsure about what any of them had to do with stress or what they meant?
- Do people react in different ways to stress?
- Is stress necessarily bad for you?
- When might it be bad for you?
- If you have some of the symptoms listed, does this necessarily mean you must be stressed?
- What are some of the ways which students have found to avoid being stressed?
- What has all this got to do with exercise?

Suggestions for follow-up work

Suggest that they make up their own wordsearches on the causes of stress (eg examinations, interviews, contests, parties). Encourage them to think of the causes of stress for other people, such as their parents, as well as for themselves. Also remind them that stress can be caused be seemingly pleasant things, like Christmas and weddings. Ask them to give their wordsearch to another pair to solve. That pair then chooses one or two of the words listed and identifies possible ways of managing the stress linked with that particular word.

SECTION 8: HEALTH-RELATED EXERCISE

ACTIVITY 72 — A stressful wordsearch

Can you find these words and terms hidden in the puzzle below? They are all signs of stress. We hope you don't find it too stressful!

AGGRESSION
ANXIETY
ASTHMA
BACK PAINS
BORED
BUTTERFLIES
DEPRESSED
DIARRHOEA
DISTRACTED
DIZZINESS

DRYNESS OF MOUTH
EAT A LOT
FORGETFUL
GUILT
HEADACHES
HIGH BLOOD PRESSURE
INDIGESTION
INSOMNIA
IRRITABLE
LACK OF APPETITE

NERVOUS
NUMB
SWEATING
TEARS
TENSION
TIREDNESS
TREMBLING
ULCERS

```
T U L D Y O X D F N T D B S L M S N E G P Y U
Y K E R S H H N U A N F I J M U W T O B R A E
H I A Y X E L O U G Y S W S O E I H O O J Q N
A T I N M A D I T R B H N V T T Z R I C D T X
B Q M E W D G S Z R X U R S E R E L L J I N E
Z A W S U A F S F O E E T P N D A U A R F L I
T E X S U C H E V O N M P T U I U C E D B Z W
T O G O J H M R D Q R A B Z E L A D T A H B T
O H P F F E C G U E F G C L C R N P T E U B Z
L R U M R S X G N O S G E E I E F I K B D R T
A R S O Q E C A K P J S R T S N R L M C B X N
T A X U J K U C S Y X S E S F R G U I Q A F Z
A I B T Z C A B N L A J I R I U N S X E S B A
E D G H J L R O A O F R M F P Z L Z G Y S E V
K Y X N H Q I K Y O N K V D N E O B E I O A L
B L S F I S A T A Y Z X W C S Z D C Z O Q T D
A B A Q N T E R U S S E R P D O O L B H G I H
N H S E E Q A D I Z Z I N E S S X M J G J J M
X X T A J A K E R T U H T X U Z N M G U N O G
I M H S U Q I Y W F C E A I N M O S N I Q C G
E L M R Q A S W D S A F E P N K X S V L E A Z
T S A E N Y S I S R V B G I J P A O U T R L Y
Y T Y Q W D W O S V N O I T S E G I D N I D T
```

210   © A Picture of Health   Permission to photocopy this page for participant use

Section 8: Health-Related Exercise

ANSWER FOR ACTIVITY SHEET 72

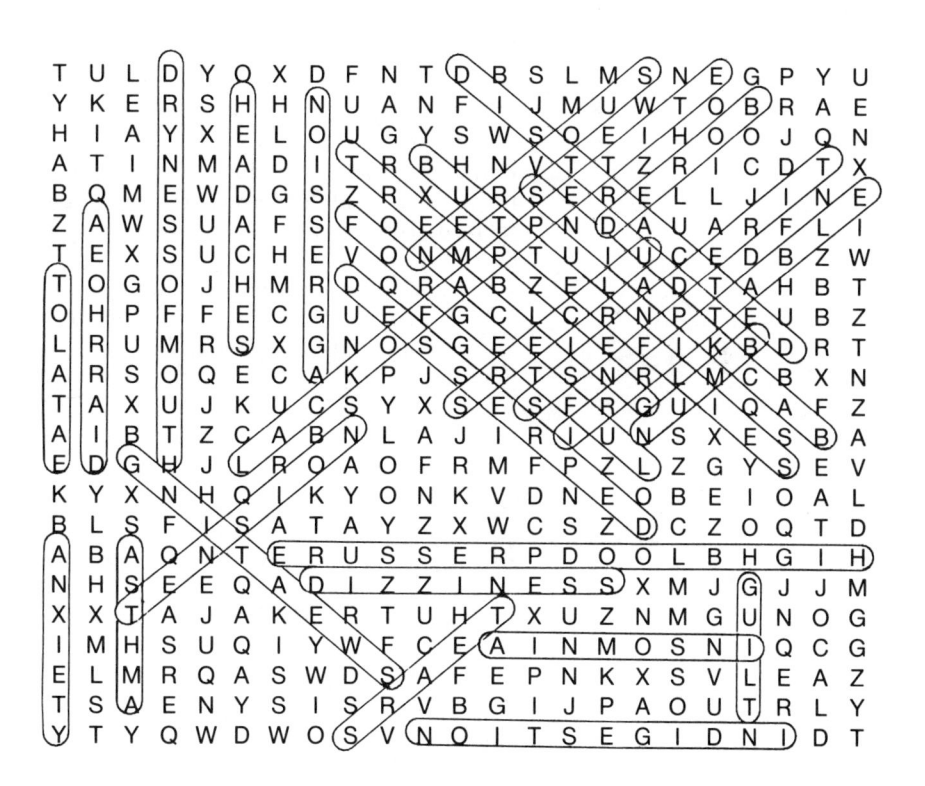

Section 8: Health-Related Exercise

Activity 73
Learning to relax

Purpose
- To help students understand the importance of relaxation
- To demonstrate some simple relaxation techniques

Time needed 20 minutes or less

What you need Pencils and paper

How you do it
1. Ask students to try this experiment. They are to hold a pencil as they would normally and write the sentence 'Tension makes it harder.' Then they should grip the pencil as hard as they can and write the sentence again. Ask them to compare the effort needed to write the sentence each way. Did they notice any changes in their breathing pattern?
2. Point out that when their body is tight or tense, they may not function as well as normal. Performance improves when they are relaxed. The following exercises all help to relieve tension. Try two or three with students.
   - Stand up and slowly stretch your right arm up as high as you can. Then bend your body to the left. Repeat, stretching your left arm and bending to the right.

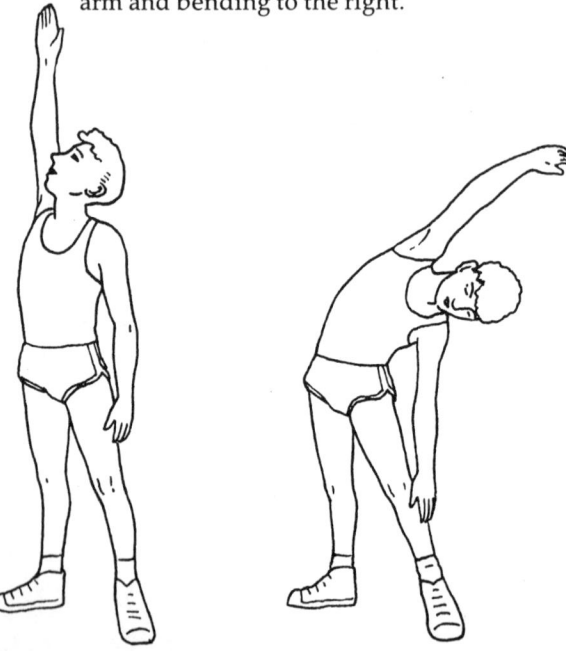

Section 8: Health-Related Exercise

- Drop your head forward. Very slowly roll it first to one side and then to the other side. Repeat until your neck muscles loosen up.
- Practise rhythmic breathing. Slowly breathe in to a count of 4, and exhale slowly to a count of 4. Do this exercise five to ten times or until you feel relaxed.
- Close your eyes. Breathe slowly. For 60 seconds or longer take yourself away from it all. Imagine you are lying on a warm beach. All you can hear is the sound of the surf.
- Beginning with your toes, tense each muscle in your body, hold for a few seconds, then relax it.
- Let your hands hang loosely at your sides. Shake one arm, then the other. Shake each leg and then shake the rest of your body. Shake each part until it feels warm.

3 Get them to discuss in the whole group how they felt doing the exercises and how they feel now.

Processing questions

- If they get tense, where in their body do they usually feel it? What happens to their breathing?
- Does anyone know any other exercises which could help people to relax?

Suggestions for follow-up work

- Arrange for someone who is trained in relaxation techniques (eg someone who teaches yoga or meditation) to take the students through a longer relaxation session.
- Brainstorm all the different ways of relieving tension students know.

SECTION 9

Personal Hygiene

SECTION 9: PERSONAL HYGIENE

ACTIVITY 74: *The hygiene game*

Purpose	• To get students to identify the personal hygiene issues which are important to different age groups
• To enable them to think of a creative way of helping people to learn about the issues
Time needed	40 minutes
What you need	Activity Sheet 74. Leaflets on hygiene from your local health promotion unit. Large pieces of paper. Coloured felt-tip pens. Large sheets of card. Magazines (optional). Scissors and gluestick. Several dice.
How you do it	1 Explain that hygiene and keeping clean are important throughout life – for health and for attractiveness, but that it can be difficult to teach about this in an interesting way.
2 Divide the class into groups of three or four. Ask each group to devise a game for a particular age group: 5–7 years, 8–10 years or 11–13 years.
It can be a card or board game. It is to help people of the age group to learn the relevant facts about hygiene and personal cleanliness. They might want to adapt well-known games; eg, snakes and ladders, and a race-track game where people get penalty and bonus cards.
3 Their first task is to decide what information the age group most needs. Give each group a copy of Activity Sheet 74 to start them thinking, and if possible other leaflets or materials on hygiene.
4 Get them to think of an imaginative way of putting that information across, and then make the game for others to try. Have a range of materials available to help with this, as listed in **What you need** above. Allow 20 minutes, although they are unlikely to have a finished product in this time.
5 Each group presents its idea for a game, explaining the basic rules and procedure.
Processing questions	• How easy was it to identify the relevant information for each age group?
• Which game do they think would be most effective for getting messages across?
• Why do they think some people don't keep themselves clean?
Suggestions for follow-up work	Finish the games and try them out, either on one another or, preferably, with the relevant age group. You could enlist the support of a local primary school and make this a longer project – with students visiting the school initially to find out how much the children already know, designing the game accordingly, trying it out with them and getting their comments.

Section 9: Personal Hygiene

The hygiene game

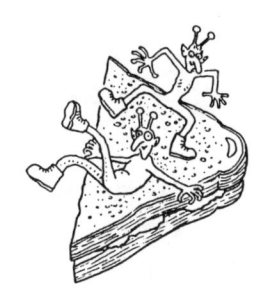

ACTIVITY SHEET 74

More than fifteen things you might need to know about keeping clean

1 GERMS Everything you touch is covered with very small living organisms. Some of these are bacteria and viruses – known as germs. If you have germs on your hands when you eat, they can get into your food and cause sickness and diarrhoea. So of all the parts of your body, your hands need washing most.

2 *Always make sure you wash your hands:*

- whenever they look, or feel dirty
- before you eat or prepare food
- after you go to the toilet
- after handling animals.

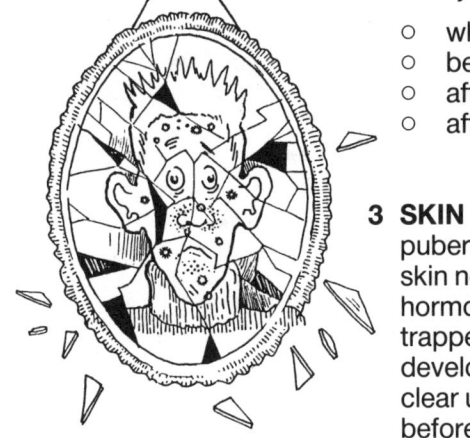

3 SKIN Because your hormones are very active during puberty, glands in your skin begin to produce more oil than your skin needs. More boys experience this than girls because male hormones cause the problem. This extra oil can become trapped in the pores of your skin and pimples or acne can develop. As your hormones settle down, your skin problems will clear up. Teenage girls may find that their skin is worse just before a period is due.

4 *Pimple problems? Six golden rules:*

- Keep skin clean – wash gently with soap. Don't rub or scrub or you could do more damage.
- Take plenty of exercise – sweating helps unblock pores.
- Don't pick spots – you can spread infection and cause scarring.
- Eat plenty of fresh fruit and vegetables – some people find chocolate and fried foods give them spots.
- Avoid thick greasy creams and make-up which can clog pores.
- Get rid of dandruff – it can make acne worse.

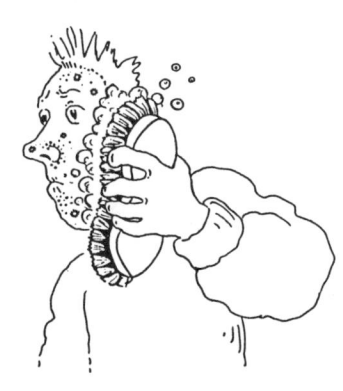

© A Picture of Health   Permission to photocopy this page for participant use

Section 9: Personal Hygiene

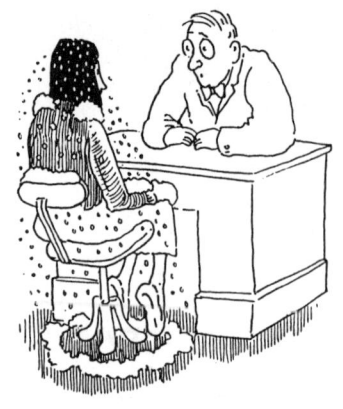

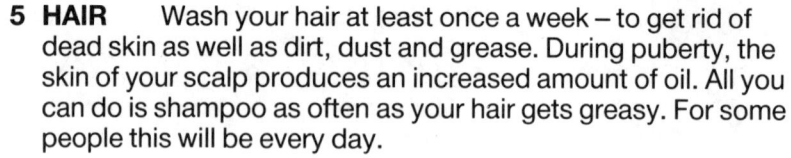

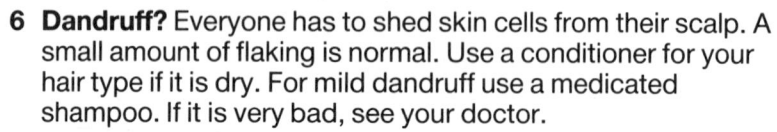

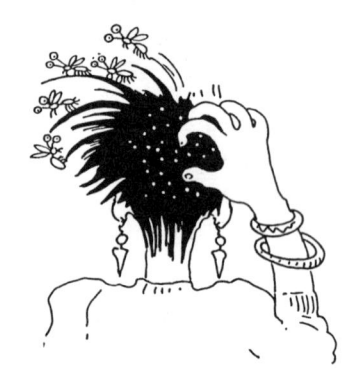

5 HAIR Wash your hair at least once a week – to get rid of dead skin as well as dirt, dust and grease. During puberty, the skin of your scalp produces an increased amount of oil. All you can do is shampoo as often as your hair gets greasy. For some people this will be every day.

6 Dandruff? Everyone has to shed skin cells from their scalp. A small amount of flaking is normal. Use a conditioner for your hair type if it is dry. For mild dandruff use a medicated shampoo. If it is very bad, see your doctor.

7 Wash your brush and comb frequently. Don't borrow or lend brushes and combs.

8 Head lice? If your head itches badly you may have caught head lice. Look carefully for the eggs or nits on your scalp. Nits are shiny and attach themselves firmly to hair. Ask your chemist or school nurse for advice about suitable treatment. This is usually a special lotion which kills the lice and nits in a few easy applications.

9 SWEAT When you get hot or excited or do some exercise, your body sweats. The sweat evaporates and you lose heat, so sweating helps the body keep itself at the right temperature.

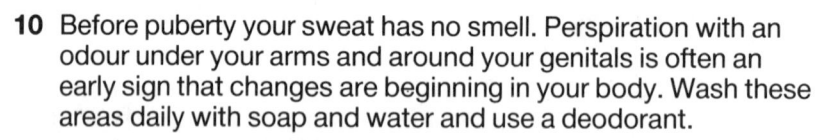

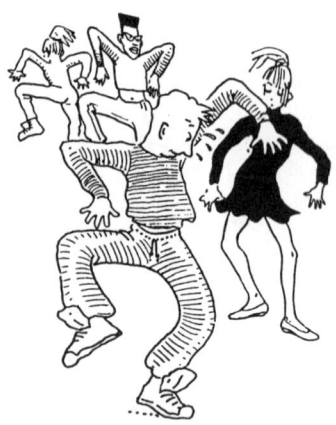

10 Before puberty your sweat has no smell. Perspiration with an odour under your arms and around your genitals is often an early sign that changes are beginning in your body. Wash these areas daily with soap and water and use a deodorant.

11 Deodorants stop sweat smelling for some hours. Anti-perspirants partially stop the sweat glands from sweating.

12 TEETH *Four golden rules:* 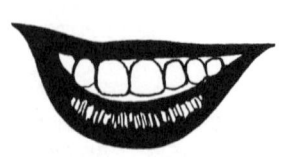
- Get rid of plaque by brushing your teeth at least once a day. Use a toothbrush with a small head and take time to clean your teeth properly, including the back teeth.
- Watch what you eat and drink. Your teeth hate sweets and you'll have problems if you're forever munching sweet things and drinking fizzy drinks between meals. Eat savoury snacks – nuts, fruit, carrots or celery.
- Toughen your teeth by using a fluoride toothpaste.
- Visit your dentist regularly – every six months.

Section 9: Personal Hygiene

13 CLOTHES   Change the clothes you wear next to your skin every single day. Wash clothes before they look dirty. Follow the care labels when washing. Outer clothes may need dry cleaning. They get smelly and dirty too. Clothes made from man-made fibres don't let the sweat evaporate as easily as cotton and wool, so you may need to change these more often. Remember that we wash clothes to get rid of smells, grease and grime, dead skin and bacteria. Dry them in the fresh air whenever you can.

14 FEET   Feet, especially ones which are still growing, need well-fitting shoes or boots. There should be growing room between your longest toe and the end of the shoe, enough width for toe wriggling, a firm fit at the heel, a straight natural inner foot shape and flexibility to let the foot muscles work.

15 *Foot care? Five golden rules:*
  o Wash feet often, at least once a day, and dry thoroughly, particularly between the toes.
  o Wear socks and tights which absorb sweat (cotton, wool or mixed fibres such as cotton/acrylic).
  o Change socks or tights every day.
  o Wash trainers inside and out regularly. Most can be washed in the washing machine.
  o Keep your toe-nails short. Cut them straight across to prevent them getting ingrown.

Section 9: Personal Hygiene

Activity 75: Problems

Purpose
- To help students find answers to problems relating to personal hygiene

Time needed 30 minutes

What you need A copy of Activity Sheet 74 for each student. Copies of Activity Sheet 75, cut up to provide one problem for each pair of pupils.

How you do it
1. Divide the class into pairs. Give each pair a problem from Activity Sheet 75. Give everyone a copy of Activity Sheet 74.
2. Ask them to imagine they are an agony aunt and write a reply to the person concerned.
3. Ask them to read out their problem and answer in the whole group.

Processing questions
- Did they have sufficient information to be able to answer the problem?
- Were the replies difficult to write?
- What other problems to do with hygiene have they come across?
- Do people have different values about cleanliness?

Suggestions for follow-up work In pairs, ask students to think of situations which they might be in where someone else has a problem with hygiene which affects them (eg you come to school with someone on the bus who smells sweaty). Ask them to write these on a card, with the question 'What would you do if . . .?' Hand this to another pair to answer. This could lead to a role play of the situation.

SECTION 9: PERSONAL HYGIENE

Problems

ACTIVITY SHEET 75

Dear Aunty,
I know that I need a deodorant. I don't want to stink of sweat. But I don't want to stink of scent either. Dad reckons that stick deodorants aren't strong enough for me. What can I do?

Dear Aunty,
My mum won't let me or my sister have a bath when we like. She says we can't afford the hot water, we've also got lodgers and have to wait our turn to use the bathroom. My friends can spend ages in the bath. It's not fair!

Dear Aunty,
How can I get rid of pimples and acne? I feel really embarrassed by them and dread people seeing my awful skin, especially when we have to get changed at school.
Please help!

Dear Aunty,
Greasy hair is my problem. Can you please tell me how to deal with it. Mum says I'll grow out of it but I need help now!

Dear Aunty,
My dad's breath really smells. It's awful! I don't really want friends round when he's in, because I get so embarrassed. What causes bad breath and what should I do about it?

Dear Aunty,
My brother had LOVE tattooed on one hand. Almost straight away he wished he hadn't. He tried rubbing salt into the skin until it bled. It was very painful. That was three months ago. He's still got the tattoo. What can he do?

Dear Aunty,
I've heard somewhere that wearing tight jeans and nylon knickers can give you an infection. Is that true?

SECTION 9: PERSONAL HYGIENE

ACTIVITY SHEET 76

What do I really need?

Purpose
- To encourage students to discuss the numerous products on the market that help people to be clean and well groomed
- To consider which are essential and for whom

Time needed 30 minutes

What you need A selection of magazines which contain advertisements for beauty/hygiene products. Scissors. Glue or gluestick. Several copies of Activity Sheet 76, if possible enlarged and cut into cards. Sheets of flipchart paper.

How you do it
1. Before the session, ask each student to bring in a women's or girls' magazine that they will not mind being cut up. Bring some yourself, in case they forget!
2. Point out that there is a wide range of toiletries on the market, often attractively packaged and advertised. Ask students to look through the magazines and cut out any products which are related to personal hygiene or being well groomed.
3. Divide the class into fairly large groups, of six to eight. Give each group a set of enlarged drawings from Activity Sheet 76; these represent a variety of products on the market to aid personal hygiene and appearance.
4. Ask each group to select twenty items from their own cuttings and the drawings.
5. Each group should hand their selection to another group, who place them face down. Each person in the group then takes it in turn to pick one up and decide whether the product shown is ESSENTIAL, USEFUL or UNNECESSARY for good personal hygiene. Once they have decided, they should ask others in the group whether they agree.
6. Ask each group to make a collage on a sheet of flipchart paper showing products in the three different categories.
7. Display these on the walls.

Processing questions
- Was it easy to find a range of products?
- How difficult was it to decide whether a product was essential, useful or unnecessary?
- Can they suggest any other products, used by their age group, which are not shown in the collages? Which category would they place them in?

SECTION 9: PERSONAL HYGIENE

Suggestions for follow-up work
- Divide the class into pairs. Give each pair a people card from Activity Sheet 52. Ask them to write a list of essential toiletries for that person. Get them to compare lists.
- Work out the costs of a range of products, as in Activity 78.

Section 9: Personal Hygiene

Activity 76 — What do I really need?

Photocopy, enlarging if possible, and cut up before use.

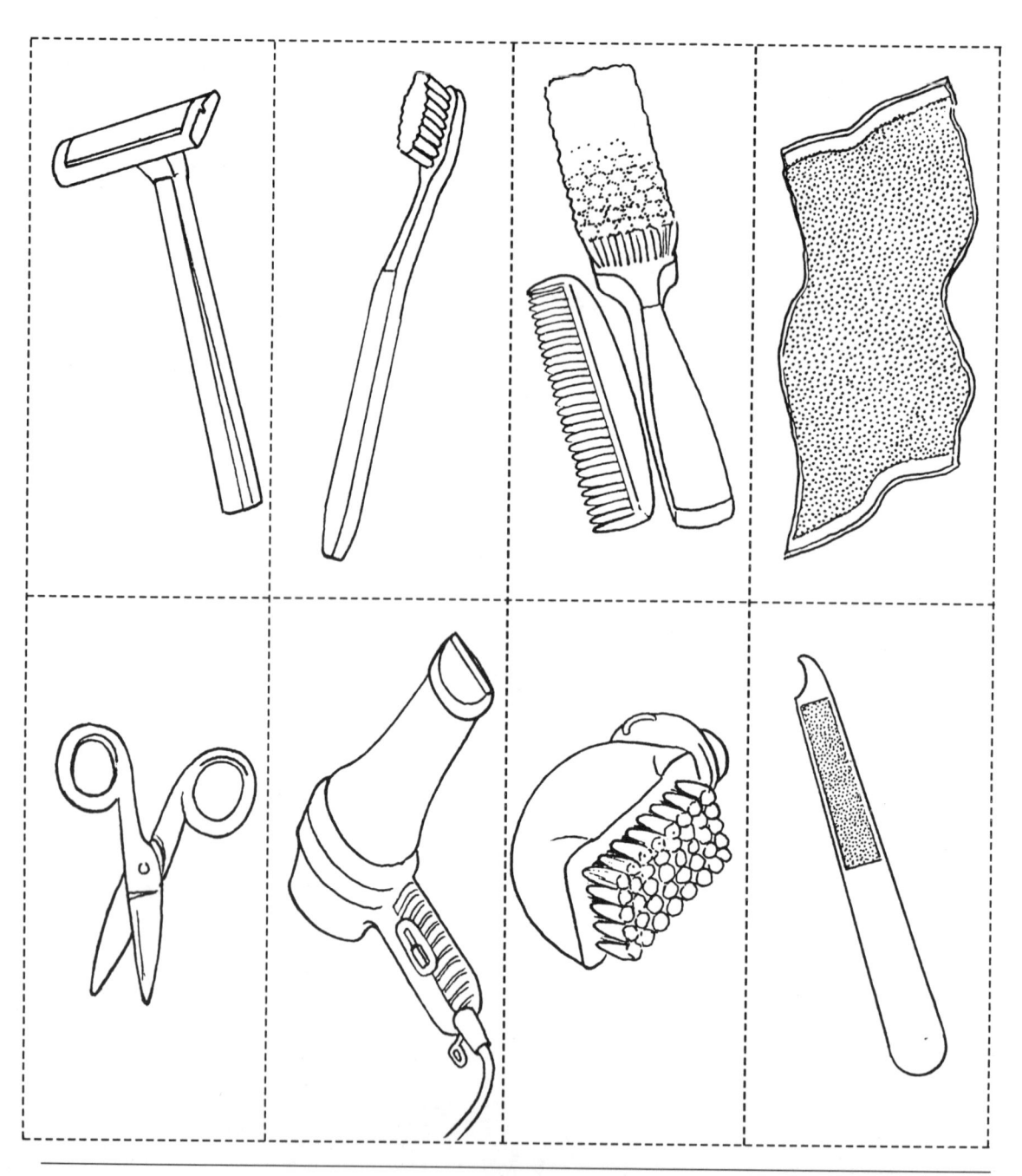

224 © A Picture of Health Permission to photocopy this page for participant use

SECTION 9: PERSONAL HYGIENE

ACTIVITY 77 — *Keeping clean*

Purpose • To explore the constraints on keeping clean

Time needed 20 minutes

What you need Several photographs/pictures from magazines of people of different ages and likely to live in different housing conditions. Blu-tack. Large sheets of flipchart paper. Pens.

How you do it
1. Divide the class into groups of four. Give each group a sheet of flipchart paper, pens and a photograph or picture.
2. Ask them to fix their photograph in the middle of the sheet. They should then write down around it all the things which could affect whether or not the person shown keeps themselves clean.

   Illustrate this with an example:
   o Whether s/he has hot water.
   o Whether s/he shares bathroom with lots of others.
   o Whether s/he cares about how s/he looks.
   o If s/he is unemployed – not many clothes.
   o If s/he is short of money – can't afford toilet things.
   o How much privacy s/he has.
3. Rotate the sheets round the groups so that students can see what others have written.

Processing questions
- Are there many words that are the same on the different sheets?
- What is the most important factor or influence on personal hygiene?
- Is it easier for some people than others?

Suggestions for follow-up work Get students to carry out a project into the living conditions of different people in the UK and other countries. How many people have easy access to hot water?

SECTION 9: PERSONAL HYGIENE

ACTIVITY SHEET 78

Counting the cost

Purpose
- To consider the cost of keeping clean
- To compare the costs in different shops and between products

Time needed About 10 minutes to set up, time after school to carry out an investigation, 20–30 minutes to discuss and display the results

What you need Copies of Activity Sheet 78 – at least as many as there are students

How you do it
1. Either brainstorm a list of products which students consider essential for personal hygiene, or use the collages and items gathered in Activity 76.
2. Divide the class into groups of three or four. Ask them to choose four items. Their task is to compare the costs of these items in three shops. Make sure that a range of products is investigated so that all groups do not choose the same four.
3. Give each group several copies of Activity Sheet 78. They need to decide who will visit which shop, to look at which products. Remember that in some large supermarkets the number of brands stocked (eg of shampoo) can be enormous. They may need to limit their research (eg to shampoo for greasy hair or frequent use).
4. Each group presents its results.

Processing questions
- How did the cost of 'own brand' products (such as Tesco or Boots) compare with other well-known brands?
- Which sizes seem best value?
- Which shops had the most choice?
- Which shops offered the best value for money?
- If you bought all the items on the essential list at once, how much would it cost?

Suggestions for follow-up work Ask students to carry out research into products which are advertised as environmentally friendly – for example, do they tend to cost more, which shops stock them, how are they environmentally friendly?

SECTION 9: PERSONAL HYGIENE

Activity 78 — Counting the cost

TYPE OF PRODUCT: ....

NAME OF SHOP: ....

Number of brands stocked: ....

Brand name	Size	Cost

TYPE OF PRODUCT: ....

NAME OF SHOP: ....

Number of brands stocked: ....

Brand name	Size	Cost

Resources

We have decided not to include a list of books and other resources as these are constantly changing. We suggest instead that you contact the Health Education Authority (the address is given in this section) who publish free of charge lists of available resources in the following areas:

AIDS
Alcohol education
Cancer education
Drugs
Family planning
Food safety
Health education for ethnic minorities
Heart disease
HIV/AIDS and sexual health
Home safety
Nutrition education
Pregnancy
Smoking education
Towards a smoke-free generation

They also produce the following annotated resource lists:

Health education resources for pupils with mild learning difficulties
Radio and TV broadcasts with relevance to health education use with young people (annual)
Relationships and sexuality: a selected resource list for professional educators of 13–18
Teaching materials for children 5–8
Teaching materials for children 9–13

Resources

Useful agencies/organisations

General

Health Education Authority
Hamilton House
Mabledon Place
London WC1H 9TX
Tel: 071 383 3833

Supplies leaflets, posters, booklets and reports on a variety of health

National Association of Young People's Counselling and Advisory Services (NAYPCAS)
Magazine Business Centre
11 Newark Street
Leicester LE1 5SS

Provides contact addresses of local services that include counselling, advice, information and befriending for young people.

Women's Health
52–54 Featherstone Street
London EC17 8RT
Tel: 071 251 6580

WHRRIC gives information on women's health issues. Wide range of publications available. Send stamped self-addressed envelope for publications list.

MIND (National Association for Mental Health)
22 Harley Street
London W1N 2ED
Tel: 071 637 0741

Works for better services for people with mental health problems, through campaigns, publications, information service, legal advice, training and education, community development and an advice service to help explain the options available to people in distress.

Tailor Made Training Ltd
240 Swanwick Lane
Lower Swanwick
Southampton SO3 7DA
Tel: 0489 576168

Offers consultancy and training in health education, experiential learning and group work, interpersonal and counselling skills, and helping people to manage change.

Drugs

Standing Conference on Drug Abuse
1–4 Hatton Place
London EC1N 8ND
Tel: 071 430 2341/2

The national co-ordinating body for voluntary organisations and agencies working in the drugs field. Publications include a national directory of services, regional lists and information affecting the drugs field. Publications list available. Twenty-four-hour freephone drug problems service giving recorded contact numbers.

TACADE
1 Hulme Place
The Crescent
Salford M5 4QA
Tel: 061 745 8925

For information, advice, training and resources on health, personal and social and, in particular, alcohol and other drug education.

The Institute for the Study of Drug Dependence (ISDD)
1–4 Hatton Place
London EC1N 8ND
Tel: 071 430 1993

Library and information service on all aspects of drug abuse.

Action on Smoking and Health (ASH)
109 Gloucester Place
London W1N 7PH
Tel: 071 935 3519

Provides information on the health effects of, and how to give up smoking. They alo provide a free information pack.

Sexuality and AIDS

Family Planning Association (FPA)
27–35 Mortimer Street
London W1N 7RJ
Tel: 071 636 7866

Has bookshop specialising in the field of sexuality. Education unit offers a professional training, education and consultation service on all aspects of personal and sexual relationships. Family Planning Information Service, at same address, provides free leaflets and fact sheets, and has library/resource room.

Brook Advisory Centre
153A East Street
London SE17 2SD
Tel: 071 708 1234/1390

Provides confidential, sympathetic advice on contraception, abortion, pregnancy and emotional and sexual problems of young people. Also produces materials.

London Lesbian and Gay Switchboard
BM Switchboard
London WC1N 3XX
Tel: 071 837 7324

Offers local, national and international information, support and advice on all aspects of gay men's and lesbians' lives (including information on HIV and AIDS).

Terrence Higgins Trust
52–54 Grays Inn Road
London WC1X 8JU
Tel: 071 242 1010 (helpline) 3–10pm
    071 831 0330 (administration)

Provides a complete range of information, education and support services to people affected by HIV and AIDS, and those caring for or working with them.

Environment

Department of the Environment
Romney House
43 Marsham Street
London SW1P 3EB
Tel: 071 276 0900

Will supply, on request, a number of free publications dealing with government principles of pollution control and legislation and the government's approach to conservation and environmental protection.

Friends of the Earth Trust
26–28 Underwood Street
London N1 7JQ
Tel: 071 490 1555

A charity committed to environmental research, education and information, currently working on issues including air, water and radioactive pollution, recycling, energy efficiency, countryside and agriculture, tropical rainforests, transport and urban environment. Publications list available on receipt of an A5 size stamped addressed envelope.

Don't forget

Your local **health promotion/education unit** (under the name of your health authority in the telephone directory) offer advice. They also have leaflets, booklets and posters on a wide variety of health issues. Materials on free loan. Details on request.
    Within your local education authority, there is also likely to be a **health education co-ordinator**, responsible for providing information and advice to schools and colleges on drugs, alcohol and AIDS.